The Veterinary Assisting Essential Book of Knowledge- *Exotics*

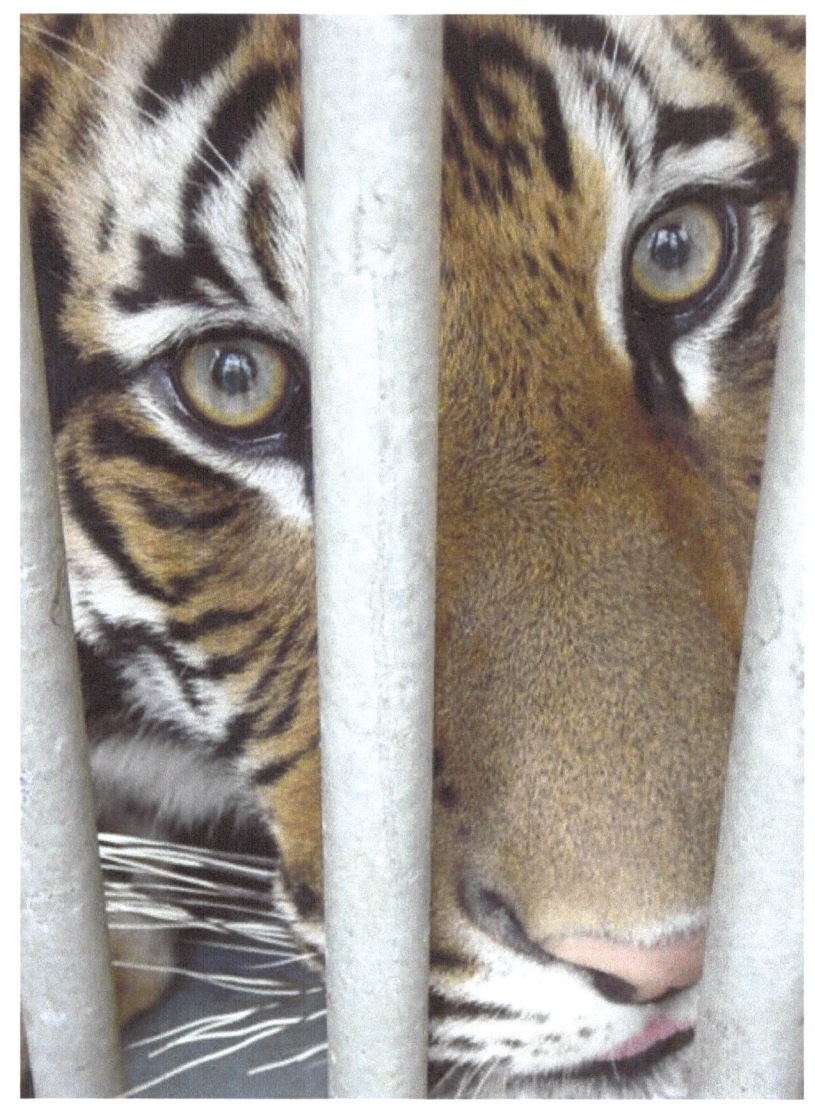

Special Thanks to my Veterinary
Assisting students
who inspire me to teach well
and who pushed me to complete this book

Table of Contents

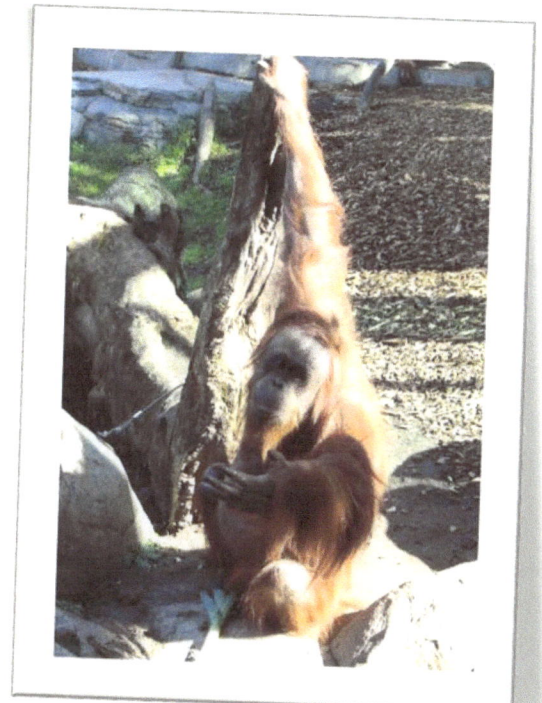

Preface

'In many cases, animals differ only by their packaging'. This self-proclaimed rationale came to me as a result of working with some of the most diverse exotic species in the world. When my career as a zoo veterinary technician began, my previous experience had been with dogs, cats and the occasional coyote or bird of prey. I quickly realized that many of the anatomical and physiological structures and processes were very similar in dogs, cats and exotics. In most cases, I was able to extrapolate what I knew about companion animals and apply it to exotics. There were, of course, some species that didn't follow the rules and required me to 'look outside the box' to determine the best strategy.

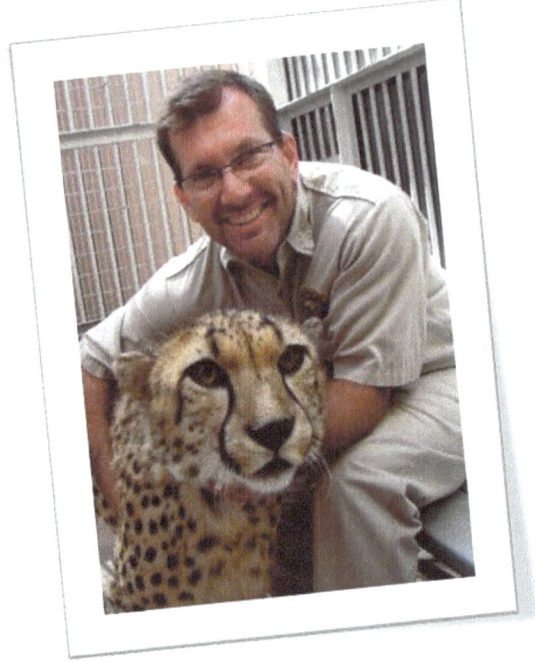

Exotic animals are some of the most amazing creatures with whom I've worked. The incredible plumage of galliformes, armored scales of pangolins, and human-like qualities of primates are qualities of exotic animals that I find so interesting; to be able to work with these animals is incredibly rewarding. Over the years I have taken hundreds of pictures of the animals I have worked with; some are shared in this book.

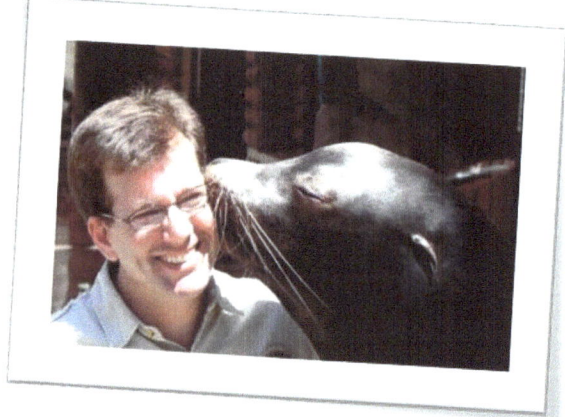

We are surrounded by wildlife; sometimes elusive, once recognized, these animals become more apparent to us. Understanding their natural behavior, medicine, nutrition and survival strategies makes us better stewards of exotic animals in captivity. My hope is that you will learn about exotic animal anatomy, physiology and husbandry, but also begin to see the amazing animals that surround us.

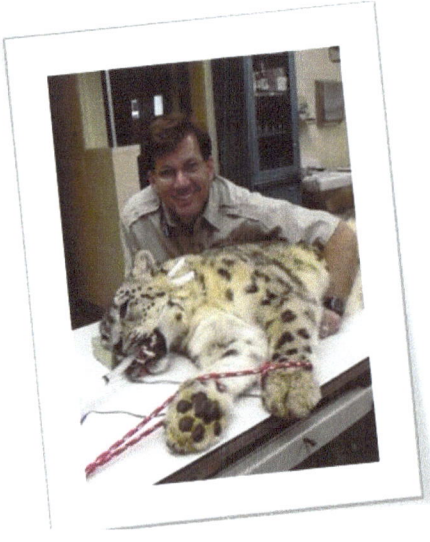

Equine Medicine

Horses have been used for thousands of years as a source of food, work, transportation, and in modern times as companions. Because of their speed and maneuverability, horses were used to herd and hunt game as well as proving useful in transporting soldiers in ancient wars. Horses proved to be stronger and faster than other working animals. The invention of the combustion engine reduced the need for horses to be used as farm implements; as a result, today, horses are more likely used for pleasure riding, performing and herding. Horse racing thoroughbreds can be worth millions of dollars and are a source of entertainment for the race track enthusiast. Police forces also use horses for crowd control and public service in areas difficult to access with vehicles. Over three-hundred breeds of horses, classified as equids, are domesticated today; these include all extant horses and ponies. The zebra is also in this family, but rarely domesticated. Equids reside in the order perrisodactyla along with Tapirs and Rhinoceroses. The term ungulate refers to all hoofed animals. All three of these families of animals have the similarity of having 'odd' numbered toes; a characteristic unique to the order perrisodactyla.

Horses, zebras, tapirs and rhinos have odd numbered toes which is a characteristic of the order perrisodactyla.

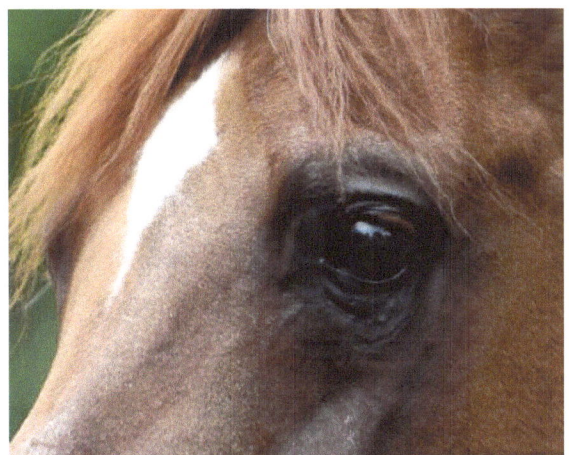

Figure 1: Horses, and other prey species, have their eyes positioned on the sides of their head

Type	Description	Example
Cold-blood	Farm or working horse, bred for strength and endurance	Percheron, Clydesdale Belgian
Hot-blood	Used for long distance riding, hot tempered	Arabian Thoroughbred
Warm-blood	Cross between hot and cold-blood	Appaloosa Morgan Quarter horse Paint horse

Table 1: Equine types and examples

Equine terminology includes technical terms as well as jargon developed over the centuries to describe horses and horse-related concepts. These terms are sometimes unique to specific countries and regions, in many cases, making the terminology highly variable.

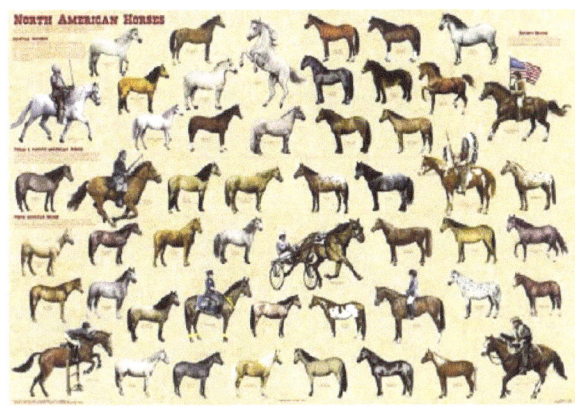

Figure 2: North American horses

Equine term	Meaning
Horse	An equid that is 14.2 hands tall or more (1 hand equals 4 inches)
Pony	An equid that is less than 14.2 hands tall
Stallion	An uncastrated male horse over 4 years of age
Colt	An uncastrated male horse less than 4 years of age
Gelding	A castrated male
Mare	Female horse over 4 years of age
Filly	Female horse less than 4 years of age
Yearling	A horse that is nearly 1 year old
Weanling	A horse that is under a year of age that has been weaned (no longer nursing)
Foal	A baby horse or pony
Halter	Headgear used to lead or tie up a horse
Bit	Mouthpiece used to help communicate with the horse; connected to reigns
Twitch	A restraint device used to calm a horse in stressful situations; it functions to squeeze the upper lip. The twitch is thought to cause the release of endorphins into the bloodstream
Saddle	The horseback riders' seat. Common types include the eastern and western saddles

Table 2: Common equine terminology

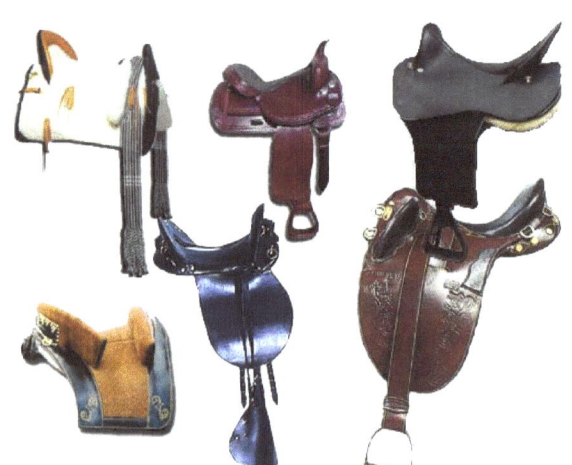

Figure 3: Saddle types used in equine riding

The Equine Veterinary Practice
The equine veterinary practice generally consists of a veterinarian and an answering service. Additionally, in most cases the veterinarian goes to the patient; this is facilitated with an ambulatory veterinary hospital in the form of a truck or van. Veterinary support staff can be less necessary in an equine practice because the client can serve to restrain their horse. The equine veterinarian may make a dozen ranch calls during the day and may be called for emergencies at night. These long hours but low overhead make equine veterinary practices lucrative businesses.

Equine Anatomy and Physiology
The skeletal anatomy of the horse is similar to that of the dog and cat. The main difference is the terminal bones of the limbs. Horses, like companion animals, walk on their fingers and toes; horse digits; however, have fused into a single terminal digit. This digit is synonymous with the middle finger on

8

the human hand. At the end of this terminal bone is the fingernail or hoof. Several terms are used to describe the bones of the horse's limb.

Common term	Equine term
Radius/ulna	Forearm
Carpus	Knee
Metacarpus	Cannon bone
Knuckle	Fetlock
First phalanx	Large pastern
Second Phalanx	Small pastern
Third phalanx	Coffin bone
Cuticle	Coronary band
Nail	Hoof

Table 3: Equine front limb terminology

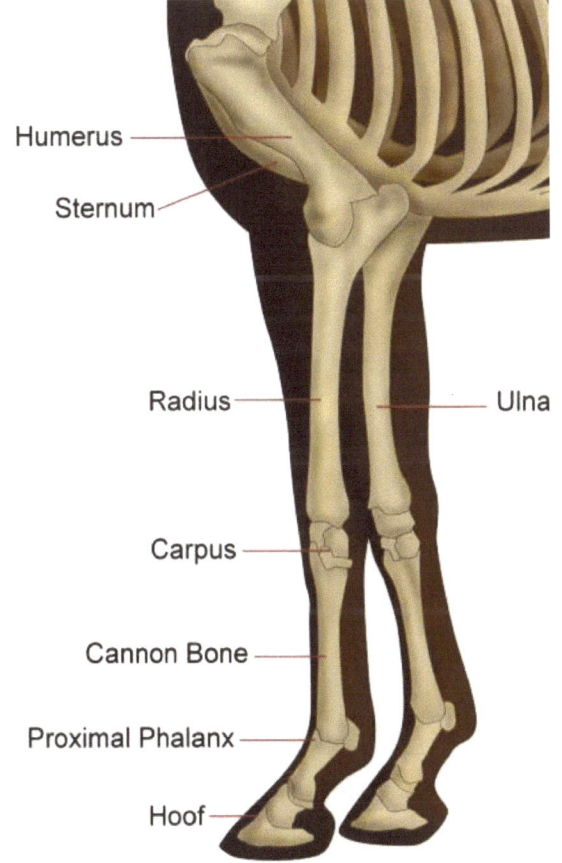

Figure 4: Skeletal anatomy of the front limbs of the horse

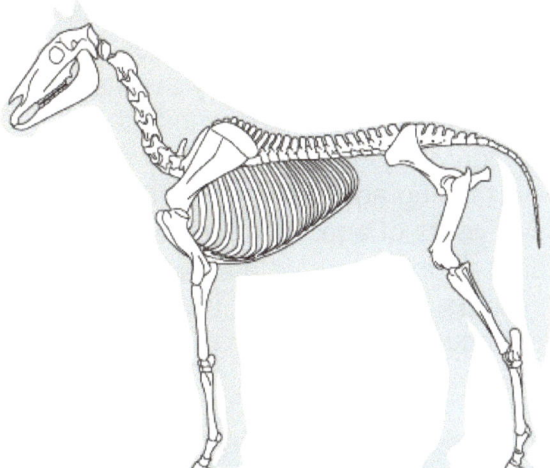

Figure 5: Skeletal anatomy of the horse

Dental Anatomy

Most herbivores, or plant eating animals, are characterized by having hypsodont dentition. These teeth are constantly erupting and being worn down by the process of chewing or mastication. The teeth are flattened with enamel folds for added strength. Animals with this type of dentition are able to pulverize plant material by grinding the material between the upper and lower arcades of teeth. Unlike dogs and cats that chew in an up-down motion, herbivores chew in a sideways motion across their flattened teeth.

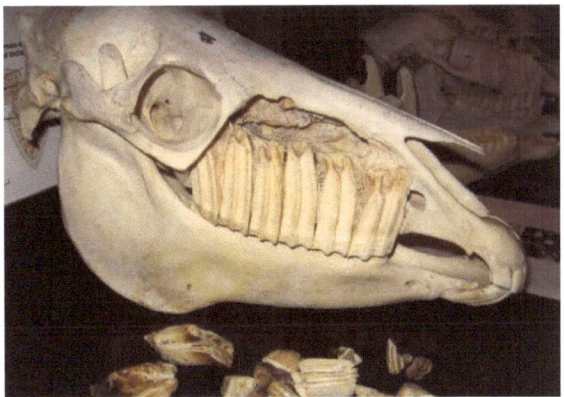

Figure 6: Equid skull showing cut-away view of maxillary dentition

Horses have deciduous or baby teeth, as well as adult teeth. Eruption and loss

9

of teeth is similar in most equids, therefore, age determination of an individual can be made by evaluation of its dentition. Most horses lose their deciduous teeth by the age of five, and start losing adult teeth at around twenty-five years of age. Male horses generally have four canine teeth between the incisors and premolars, and may or may not have four wolf teeth or vestigial premolars.

Type	Numbers Female	Numbers Male
Incisors	12	12
Canines	0-4	4
Wolf	0-4	0-4
Premolars	12	12
Molars	12	12
Total Deciduous	24	24
Total Adult	36	40

Table 4: Equine teeth types and numbers

Circulatory System

Like all mammals, the horse heart contains four chambers, two paired atria, and two ventricles. The physiology and function of the system is no different than a dog or cat; the larger the species, the larger the size of the heart. The equid heart weighs approximately 4.5 kilograms (10 pounds). This is necessary to pump the nearly 52 liters (13.2 gallons) of blood throughout the horse's body.

If you know the anatomy and physiology of a dog heart, you know all there is to know about a horse heart, and your own heart for that matter.

Respiratory System

Like all mammals, the horse respiratory system functions as a place of oxygen and carbon dioxide exchange. The diaphragm drives respiration by its muscular contraction causing inhalation; relaxation of the diaphragm causes exhalation. The lung capacity, referred to as the tidal volume, is between five and ten liters. This is compared to a human tidal volume of one to two liters. Horses are in a group of animals called obligate nasal breathers. During normal respiration, the epiglottis occludes the oropharynx. The position of the epiglottis forces air through the nasal passages during respiration. Swelling or obstruction of the nasal passages can be life-threatening for an obligate nasal breather.

Digestive System

Digestion of plant material is a challenging task. Herbivores spend a great deal of time acquiring, chewing and digesting plant material in order to obtain required nutrition. The breaking down of plants into useable energy involves the extraction of useable glucose from cellulose. In herbivores this process is further aided by bacterial fermentation in the digestive tract.

The process of digestion starts (like dogs) in the mouth where plant material is broken down into a slurry with the aid of saliva. Having ample water available is important in herbivore digestion.

This slurry or digesta, makes its way to the stomach where acids continue the digestion process. Horses are considered monogastric, having a single chambered simple stomach, and are unable to vomit or belch.

Most digestion occurs in the intestines of horses. Bacteria help break down plant material in a process called fermentation; the byproduct of this process is methane gas production. Horses and other hind-gut fermenters tend to be flatulent for this reason. The cecum (similar to the appendix in humans), is an important and prominent location for bacterial fermentation. Because fermentation occurs primarily in the intestines, horses are referred to as hind-gut fermenters. Unfortunately, this is not a highly efficient process and much of the nutrients and plant material are lost in the feces. Horse feces are heavily laden with undigested plant material. Horses and other hind-gut fermenters must eat large volumes of food to obtain necessary nutritional calories.

Colic refers to any digestive pain or discomfort experienced by horses. Colic is characterized by inappetence, stretching, pawing the ground, pacing and rolling on the ground. Causes of colic include: food, sand or enterolith impaction, gas buildup, endoparasites and gastric torsion. Treatment may include analgesics or may require surgery. Colic can be life-threatening.

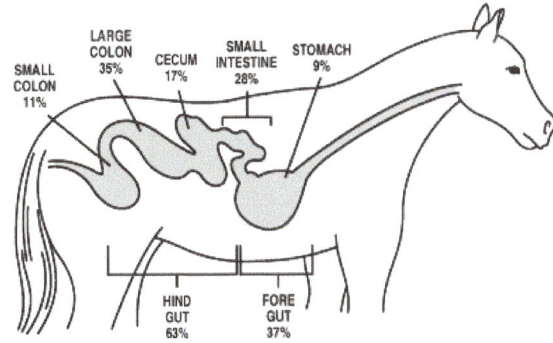
Figure 7: Equine digestive anatomy

Restraint Types

Horse restraint is necessary to perform most veterinary medical procedures. These large animals can easily injure handlers and veterinary staff if not properly restrained. The method of restraint is usually dictated by the procedure being attempted as well as the temperament of the patient. In some cases, the horse owner is the best

person to restrain their horse, and in other cases, they can be the worst. The halter is the most convenient restraint device for the horse. It is the least invasive, but exceptionally effective at containing a tractable horse. The halter fits over the head of the horse and may include a mouth bit. A rope attached to the halter gives handlers substantial control of the horse's head.

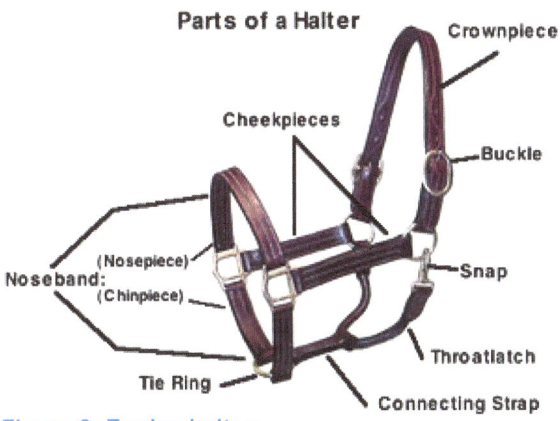
Figure 8: Equine halter

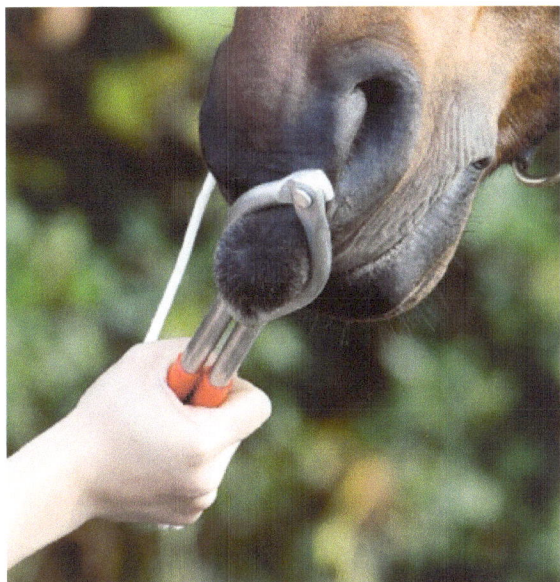
Figure 9: Equine twitch

11

A twitch makes use of the natural endorphin release that prey species have when being attacked by a predator. By pinching the skin, or lip of a horse, the endorphin release causes a calming effect on the animal, much like that caused when scruffing a cat. A twitch is a metal device that can be placed on the horses lip, and left on for a limited amount of time. Twitches may be effective for short procedures where patient movement needs to be minimized.

A chute may be necessary to restrain a fractious horse; the walls of a chute protect the handler from potential kicking by the horse. Horse kicks are a significant concern for the veterinary staff, and can lead to serious injury.

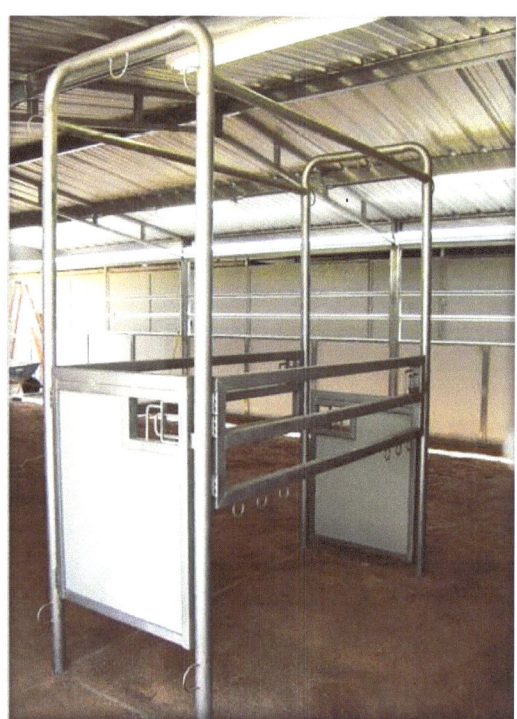

Figure 10: Large animal containment chute

Chemical restraint on horses may be necessary in some veterinary medical procedures. Dental and hoof care may require sedatives and anesthetics to facilitate the procedures. Sedatives and anesthetics are usually given at minimal doses to maintain the horse in an upright position. This is often termed a standing sedation, and generally results in fewer anesthetic related complications.

Physical Exam

As with companion animals, the physical exam of a horse should be sequential so no portion of the exam is inadvertently missed. It is generally best to start the exam, as with dogs and cats, at the head. Disposition and behavior can be determined from the front of the horse, and the head is generally restrained. Horses have two blind spots, one directly in front of them and one behind them, so approaching a horse should be made from the side. Additionally, horses tend to be more familiar with being approached from their left side, as this is the side that riders usually mount them. The physical exam of the horse is not unlike that of the dog and cat; they all have many of the same parts in the same locations. Several things are not like dogs and cats and should be included in the physical exam.

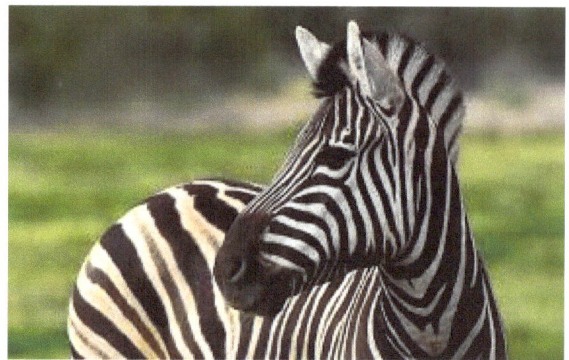

Figure 11: Domestic horses and asses are related to the three species of zebra; the Grevy's, Mountain and Plains Zebras

Evaluation	Why it's Checked
Dental Check	Horses' teeth are constantly erupting; improper wear can lead to jaw pain, improper chewing, and digestion problems.
Hoof Check	Horses walk on their toes; improper hoof wear or alignment can lead to pain and lameness.
Gut Check	Horses have a lot of guts; digestive noises or gut sounds can indicate sand impaction or digestive pain. A stethoscope can be used to listen for gut sounds.
Hydration Check	Horses do not have as much subcutaneous (SQ) space as dogs and cats; squeezing the eyelid is one way to determine hydration in the horse.
Temperature	Hyperthermia can indicate infection; a rectal temperature is generally used, but due to the size of the rectum, care should be taken to get the temperature of the wall of the rectum and not the feces. The normal temperature of the horse is 99-101 degrees Fahrenheit.
Pulse	Horses have a large chest; it may be difficult to listen to the heart rate of a horse, so the pulse rate can be determined using the femoral, brachial or facial arteries. The normal pulse rate in the horse is 36-42 beats per minute.
Respiration	Horses breathe at a much slower rate than smaller animals; respiration rate can be determined by looking for abdominal movement or watching the nares flare during breaths. The normal respiration rate in horses is 8-12 breaths per minute.

Table 5: Common equine veterinary assessments

Injection Sites

Due to their large size, horses can be easily injected with parenteral medications. Injection techniques used with companion animals are applicable with horses; always aspirate the syringe prior to injection. Even though they are large, horses will sometimes respond to the needle when injected; lightly hitting the injection site prior to administration may reduce the horse's response to the needle. In some cases, inserting the needle alone, then connecting the syringe to it, can be an effective way to eliminate having a dangling syringe in the horse if it moves or reacts. Caution should always be taken when giving injections in or near the rear limbs, as a horse may kick when injected.

Subcutaneous injections (SQ) can be given in the areas around the base of the neck or in any of the spaces around the limbs. The interscapular region has limited SQ space. There is significantly less SQ space in a horse when compared to that of a dog or cat.

Intramuscular injections (IM) can be given in any of the limbs of the horse, but the muscular neck tends to be safer and more convenient.

Intravenous injections (IV) can be administered in the cephalic, saphenous or jugular veins as in companion animals. The jugular veins in horses are quite large and conveniently accessible in the jugular furrow of the neck. The jugular veins in the horse are about the size of a garden hose.

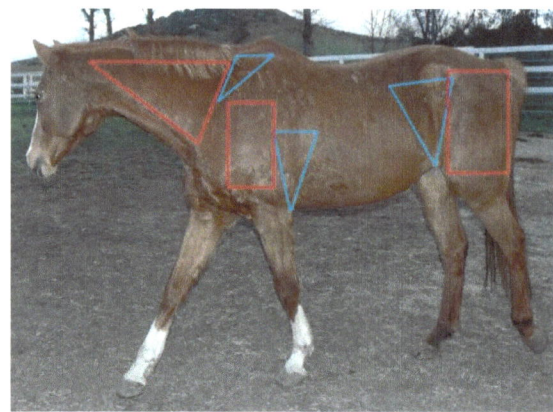

Figure 12: Equine subcutaneous injection sites (blue) and intramuscular injection sites (red)

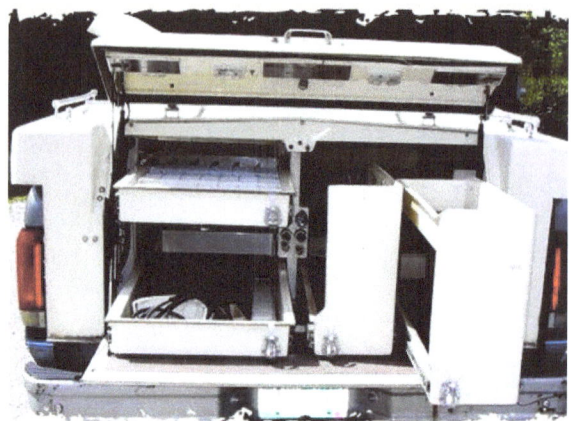

Figure 13: The equine ambulatory vet truck contains compartments for needed veterinary equipment

Preventative Medicine

Veterinary care is necessary for dogs, cats and horses. The main difference is that instead of bringing your horse to the veterinarian, most veterinarians must go to the horse. Equine veterinarians typically have vehicles for offices; they are ambulatory veterinary clinics on wheels.

Vaccinations are designed to protect horses from serious diseases. Passive transfer of antibodies occurs during nursing; colostrum is transferred to the foal in the mother's milk. Passive transfer and the process of vaccination and active transfer are similar to those for the dog and cat.

Vaccination	Disease	Frequency
Rabies	Fatal viral neurologic disease	Annual
Tetanus	An anaerobic bacterial disease	Annual
EEE/WEE	Eastern and western equine encephalomyelitis; transmitted by mosquitoes.	Annual
West Nile	Mosquito vectored disease causing encephalitis; the horse is a dead-end host.	Annual

Table 5: Core vaccines for the horse

Most endoparasites have life-cycles that at some point are spent on the ground. Animals that feed from the ground, therefore, are more susceptible to parasite ingestion and infection. Most horses are placed on prophylactic deworming medications due to their increased risk of infection. Depending on the medication used, deworming products are administered in eight to twelve week intervals. Endoparasites frequently seen in horses include ascarids, tapeworms and strongyles.

Dental care is an important aspect of equine preventative medicine. Dental health is necessary for proper feeding and digestion; dental problems can be tied to lameness. The most common procedure performed on horses teeth is called 'floating'. A rasp is used to file

14

down the surface of the teeth; the removal of points and high spots enables the upper and lower teeth to articulate properly for mastication. Sharp points and malocclusions can lead to pain and improper digestion of food. Dental floating may need to be performed annually or more frequently depending on the horse. In many cases, sedation is required to properly facilitate a dental floating on a horse.

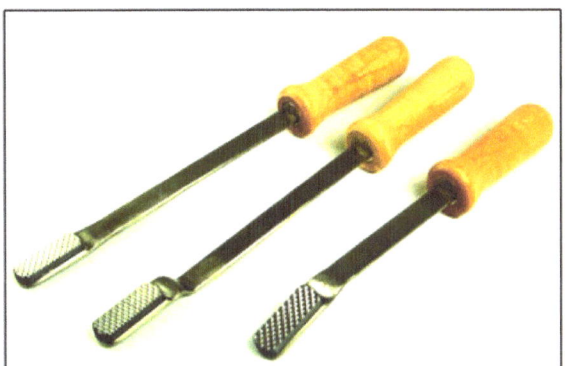

Figure 14: Equine dental floating tools

Hoof care is an essential component of horse care. Hoof problems and associated lameness are a common reason for a veterinary visit. Lameness can be a serious and difficult problem to treat; causes include improper hoof wear, sprain, excessive weight, infection and trauma.

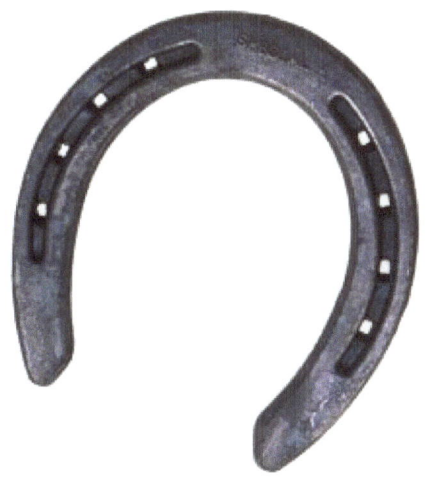

Figure 15: Metal horse shoe and nail holes

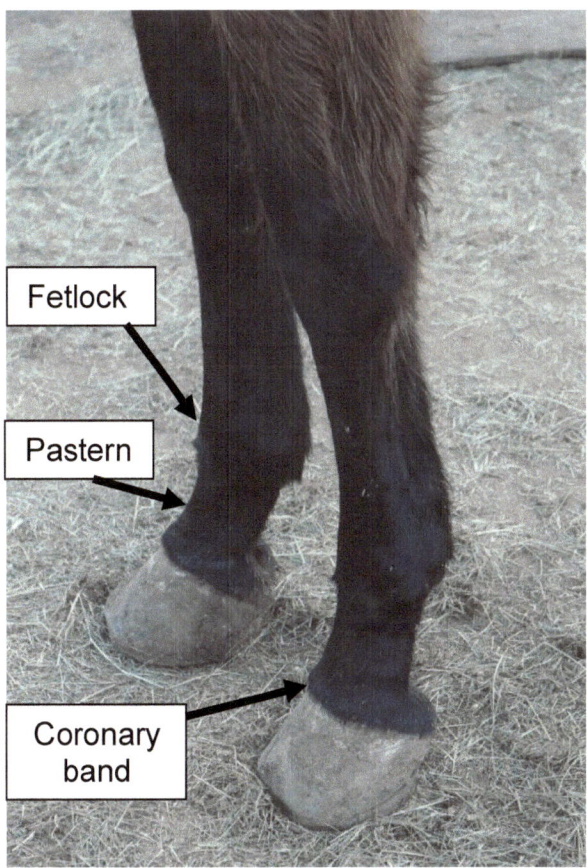

Figure 16: The horse hoof and limb

Term	Explanation
Laminitis	Inflammation of the lamina resulting in the separation of the hoof from the coffin bone.
Founder	Laminitis that results in the coffin bone detaching and sinking through the bottom of the sole. Founder is a maritime term meaning 'to sink'.
Farrier	Person who specializes in hoof care, trimming, balancing and placing shoes on their hooves.
Shoe	A U-shaped metal shoe used to protect a horse's foot from wear and tear. Shoes are placed on domestic horses because of abnormal wear, substrates, and activity differences from their wild counterparts.

Table 6: Equine foot terminology

15

Imaging

The most common imaging utilized in equine medicine includes radiography and ultrasonography. Both modalities are diagnostically valuable, and are compact and portable for the ambulatory practitioner. Most radiographic studies are focused on the limbs and hooves, while ultrasound is a valuable tool in fertility and artificial insemination procedures.

Radiography

Portable radiography systems enable equine veterinarians the ability to take radiographs 'in the field'. Portable x-ray machines are not as powerful as larger hospital units, but are able to penetrate the limbs of the equine patient. Digital sensor panels and software allow for the immediate viewing of radiographs 'in the field'. Due to the frequency of lameness, radiography is an important and valuable diagnostic tool for the equine veterinarian called upon to examine and diagnose in the field.

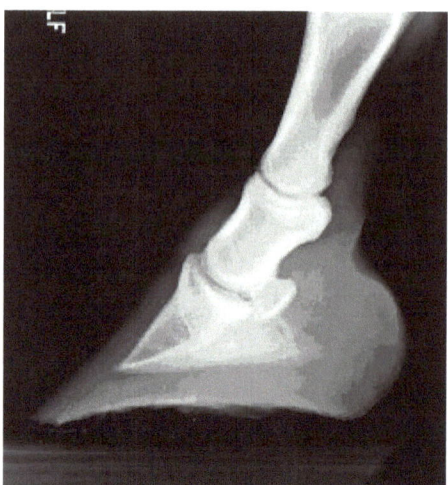
Figure18: Lateral hoof radiograph of the horse

Ultrasound

Portable ultrasound units can be used in the field to evaluate conditions relating to patient lameness and reproductive status. The ultrasound is useful in determining follicular development, ovulation and fetal development in horses that are in natural or artificial insemination breeding programs. The status of follicular development is essential for artificial insemination. The ultrasound can find fluid in joints, evaluate the quality of heart function and identify objects like uroliths in the gut of equids.

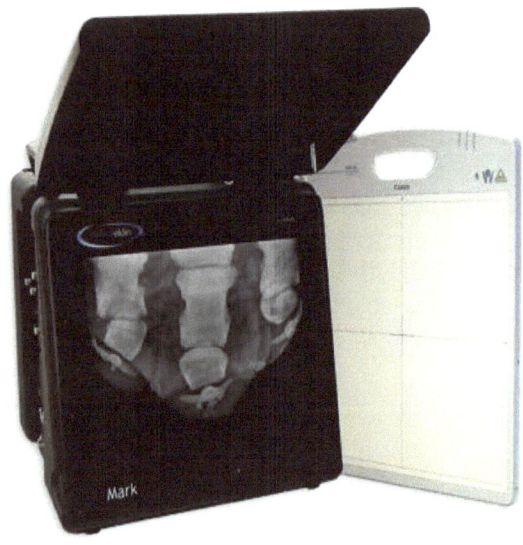
Figure 17: Portable digital radiography viewer and plate

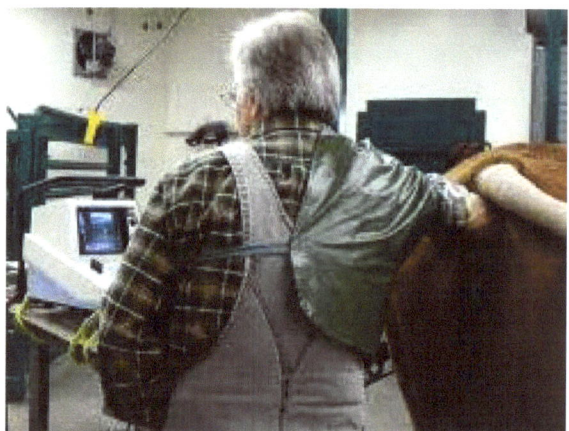
Figure 12: Reproductive ultrasound of the horse; the probe is inserted rectally

16

Medical Diseases

Horses are susceptible to a variety of diseases. Just like any species, these diseases can be spread by direct contact, blood and other fluids, feces, the environment or by vectors such as flies, ticks and mosquitoes. Vaccines are available for many common equine diseases; however, some diseases are more difficult from which to protect. West Nile virus, a disease that originated in Africa, caused significant mortality in horses until the advent of an effective vaccine. Other diseases, such as dryland distemper, are thought to be seasonal and spread by flies during the warmer months of the year.

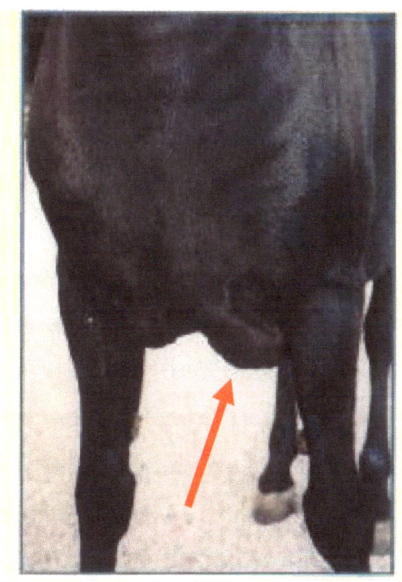

Figure 20: Dryland Distemper (aka. pigeon fever) abscesses in the breast of the horse

Disease	Causative agent	Symptoms	Treatment
Dryland Distemper aka. Pigeon Fever	Bacterium Corynebacterium pseudotuberculosis	Abscesses of the chest and midline, lameness, lethargy, fever and weight loss	Draining of abscesses, antibiotics and pain management
Strangles aka. Shipping Fever	Bacterium Streptococcus equi	Fever, poor appetite and depression followed by nasal discharge and abscesses of the lymph nodes	Isolation from other horses, drain abscesses, antibiotics if early stages (a vaccine is available)
West Nile Virus	Mosquito-borne virus	Encephalitis and meningitis, ataxia, fever, dullness and seizures	No specific treatment; horses are dead-end hosts. (a vaccine is available)
Tetanus aka. Lockjaw	anaerobic bacterial disease	colic and stiffness, spasms in the jaw, neck and hind legs	Draining of the wound, antibiotics (a vaccine is available)
Equine herpesvirus aka. Rhinopneumonitis	Viral disease	Respiratory disease symptoms including fever, cough and nasal discharge, also causes abortion	Supportive care, antiviral drugs in some cases (a vaccine is available)
Potomac Horse Fever	Arthropod vectored bacterial disease	High fever, lethargy, loss of appetite and diarrhea	Antibiotics and fluid therapy(a vaccine is available but its efficacy is questionable)

Table 7: Common equine diseases

Feeding and Nutrition

Horses are fed both hay and grain, ideally several times each day to maintain ideal digestion. Generally five to ten pounds of grain concentrates and approximately ten to twenty pounds of hay (1% to 2% of the horse's bodyweight) are fed daily. Hay or roughage should serve as the bulk of a horse's caloric intake. Roughage is important to the equine digestive process. Types of hay include Alfalfa, Timothy, Orchard grass, Bermuda, Oat and Straw.

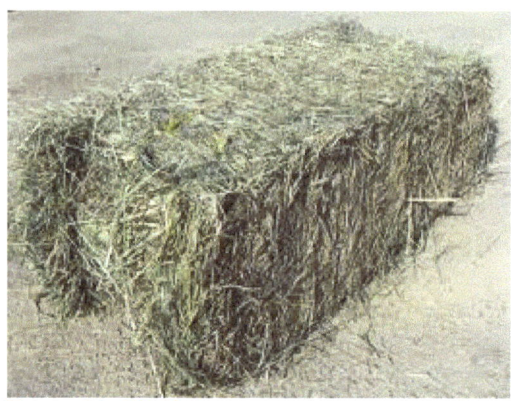
Figure 21: Alfalfa hay

Salt is an essential component of a horse's diet and is generally provided in the form of a salt lick.
Horses consume about ten gallons of water daily; water should be available at all times.

Neonatal Care

Most prey animals have a very efficient birthing process. In the wild it is important for the newborn to deliver quickly and begin walking immediately. Once ambulatory, most neonates begin nursing from their mother. This process is common for both wild and domesticated prey animals. Sometimes, however, new mothers fail to provide the

assistance and experience so their offspring fail to thrive. In these cases, intervention may be necessary. Most neonate domestic equids can be easily bottle-fed in the absence of an attentive mother. If natural nursing never occurred, then there was likely no transfer of maternal antibodies in the form of first milk or colostrum. In these cases, plasma transfusions from adult donor animals may be indicated.

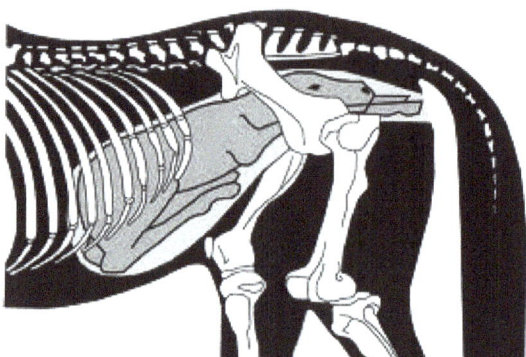
Figure 22: Normal pre-delivery positioning of the foal

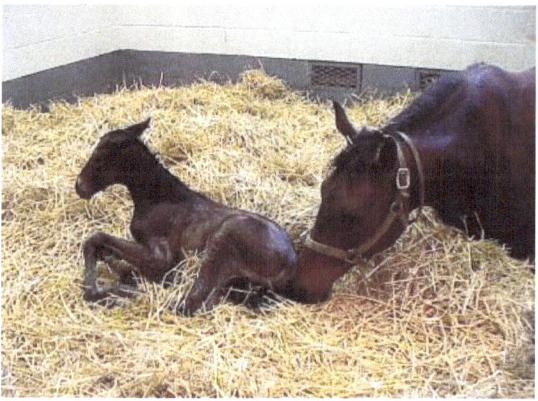
Figure 23: Post-parturition of the horse

Anesthesia

Anesthesia, and more commonly sedation, is used to facilitate procedures on equids. A 'standing sedation' describes the process of immobilizing an equid without causing them to lose their ability to remain upright. By using this strategy, anesthetic risks can be

18

minimized. Sedatives are often administered intravenously in the jugular vein which produces immediate effects. A standing sedation can be easily performed in a barn, yard or corral; this is a convenient way to facilitate medical care without transporting the patient to a veterinary hospital.

Reasons for a standing sedation can include:

      Wound care and treatment
      Laceration closure
      Dental teeth floating
      Hoof trimming and shoeing
      Artificial insemination

Common anesthetics and sedatives used in equids include:

      Ketamine
      Zylazine
      Detomidine
      Carfentanil
      Etorphine

Drugs used for standing sedation usually produce short term effects, and in some cases can be reversed with an appropriate antagonist.

> Standing sedation is useful for minor procedures and can be done in the field.

Surgery

If general anesthesia for surgery is required, equids should be transported to a proper veterinary facility, intubated and maintained on a large animal anesthetic breathing circuit. A typical horse may require a twenty millimeter endotracheal tube; a typical domestic cat requires a four millimeter tube. The gas anesthetic, Isoflurane, is commonly used to maintain these patient's at a

surgical level of anesthesia. Mechanical ventilation may be necessary if respiration quality decreases and expired carbon dioxide levels become elevated.

Surgical procedures may include invasive procedures such as abdominal exploration, orthopedic repair or reproductive intervention (dystocia).

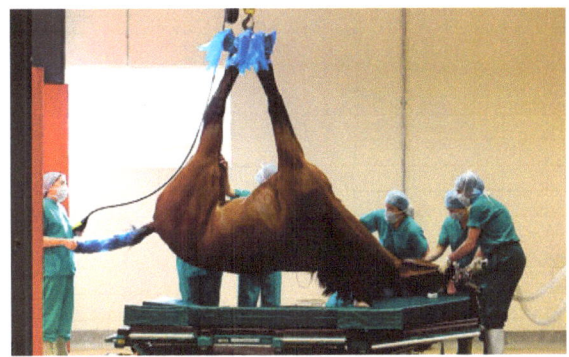

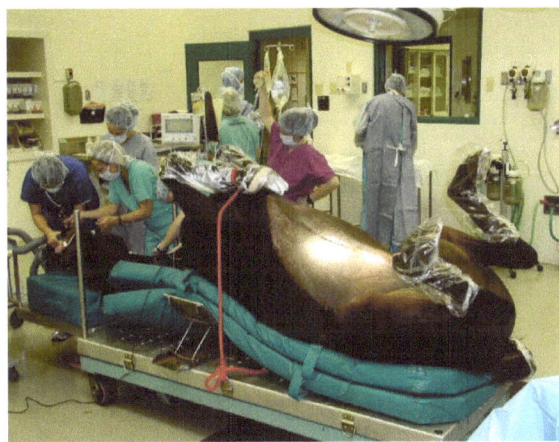

Figure 24: Equine surgical procedure hoisting (top), and positioning.

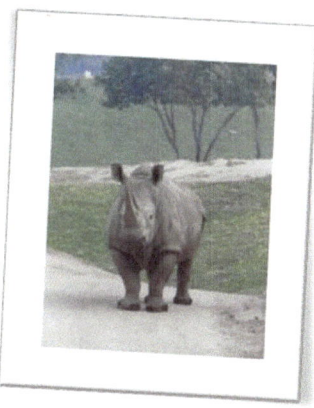

White Rhinoceros

19

Livestock Medicine

Livestock are considered animals used as a commodity of food, work or textiles. These hoofed animals, also called ungulates, are generally domesticated and are housed in a 'herd' agricultural setting. Types of livestock include goats, sheep, cattle, swine, llamas, camels, buffalo and deer.

Livestock Terminology

Many of the terms used to describe horses' anatomy and physiology can be used for livestock. The main difference between horses and livestock is the digestive anatomy; most significant is the multi-chambered stomach. Nearly all livestock, except for swine, are considered ruminants, and are characterized by the process of rumination or re-chewing their food. Terms related to livestock are as follows:

Term	Definition
Livestock	A group of animals used for food, work or textiles; most are artiodactyls with a ruminant digestive system. Sometimes referred to as 'beasts of burden'
Ungulate	Any hoofed mammal
Ruminant	Latin word meaning to chew over again
Foregut Fermentation	Digestive process where bacterial breakdown of plant material occurs-the foregut is the front part of the digestive tract
Cud	Semi-chewed food that has been regurgitated so it can be further chewed

Table 8: Livestock terms

The Livestock Veterinary Practice

The livestock veterinary practice functions similarly to that of an equine practice; they are typically ambulatory practices. Because these animals are considered commodities more than companions, there may be less investment in their individual veterinary care. In large livestock farms, animals may be culled because of illness rather than treated; it would be cost prohibited to treat individuals. Herd management techniques such as providing quality feed and prophylactic medicine for all individuals is often utilized, realizing that a fraction of the animals will not maintain health. Individuals who own a single animal or small herd may devote more money and resources to their animals' veterinary health.

Livestock Anatomy and Physiology

Anatomically, a cow is similar in structure to a horse; many of the bones are the same. An easily discernible characteristic of most livestock resides in their feet. Whereas equids have 'odd' numbered toes, most livestock are characterized by having 'even' numbered toes. These animals are classified as artiodactyls, and are sometimes referred to as 'cloven hoofed' animals.

Ruminants, also called cloven hooved animals, have even numbered toes.

One of the most significant physiological characteristics of livestock is their unique gastro-intestinal system. Just as with horses, livestock digestion begins with the chewing of plant material in the mouth. Once food is swallowed, it proceeds to the stomach. Unlike horses, most livestock have a complex four-chambered stomach in which most breakdown of food occurs. This group of animals is referred to as foregut fermenters. Furthermore, livestock often can be seen re-chewing their food, sometimes called cud, as part of a process called rumination. Most livestock, therefore, are able to regurgitate their food in the form of cud and commonly belch due to gas produced by stomach fermentation.

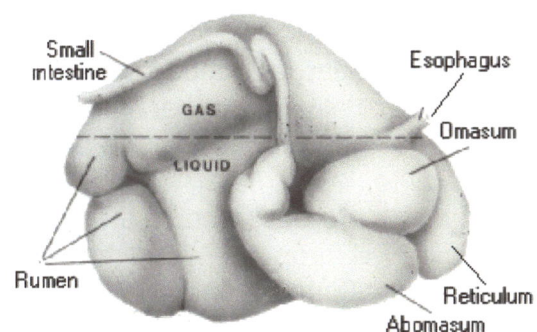

Figure 13: Anatomy of the ruminant stomach

Ironically, the first chamber of the ruminant stomach is called the rumen.

Here, food is mixed with saliva and separated into a fluid portion and solid mass called cud or bolus. This material is regurgitated and re-chewed to further break it down and mix with additional saliva. The second chamber, called the reticulum, is similar to the rumen and aids in the breakdown and fermentation of the food. The third chamber, called the omasum, receives the liquid digesta; here, water and many inorganic nutrients are absorbed into the bloodstream. The final chamber, called the abomasum is considered the true stomach. Digestive processes similar to other animals occur here. Digesta leaves the stomach and enters the small intestine where most nutrient absorption occurs. Additional fermentation occurs in the cecum and large intestine.

Livestock, like horses, have hypsodont dentition characterized by the constant eruption and wearing of the teeth. This group of animals usually lacks upper incisors; they instead have a thick dental pad on the roof of their mouth.

Ruminant livestock are called foregut fermenters, and are characterized by having a multi-chambered stomach where most of the breakdown of food occurs.

Physical Exam

The process of a physical exam for livestock is similar to that of any animal. The importance of having an exam sequence cannot be understated. By examining patients with the same sequence and methods, exams will be thorough and complete. Large patients may require different restraint methods than a smaller companion animal.

Eyes, ears, nose and throat:
Look for discharge, weeping, swelling, redness or injury.
Limbs and hooves:
Look for lameness, swelling or overgrowth.
Heart and lungs:
Determine heart and respiration rate. Listen for heart murmurs and respiratory noises. This may be difficult to assess on very large patients.
Coat:
Evaluate quality of coat and fur. Look for hair loss and injuries.
Hydration:
Evaluate hydration status; many species of livestock do not have an interscapular 'scruff' area like companion animals. Hydration may be determined by pinching the eyelid and assessing its elasticity.
Umbilicus:
Especially in neonates, the umbilicus should be inspected for redness or herniation.
Reproductive:
Look for abnormal discharge, blood or swelling of the genitalia.

Injection Method	Location
Subcutaneous (SQ)	The flanks, especially around the axillary and inguinal regions.
Intramuscular (IM)	The limbs, and neck in larger patients. Be cautious of the hind limbs due to kicking.
Intravenous (IV)	The jugular veins or tail vein.

Table 9: Injection types and sites for livestock

Restraint

Restraint of livestock is generally based on the size of the animal. Smaller goats and pigs may be restrained manually, while larger sheep and cattle may need additional equipment.
A chute is a common way to limit an animal's ability to move, and therefore facilitate effective restraint. In the dairy industry, for example, cows are placed in a chute so they can be safely milked.

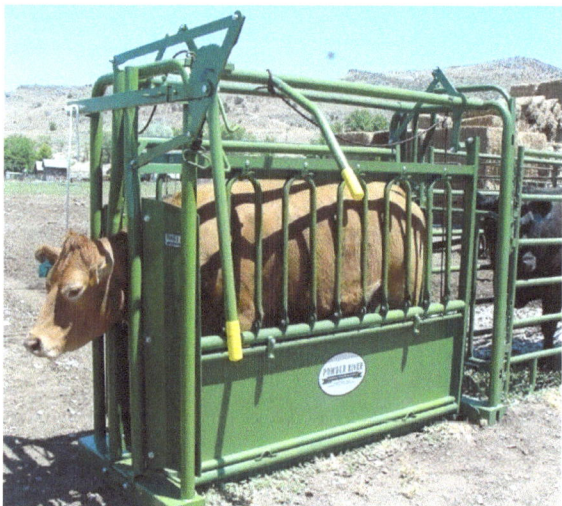

Figure 14: Livestock chute (image from ValleyVet.com)

A tamer is useful when complete immobilization is needed. A tamer makes use of the general ungulate body conformation to facilitate restraint. Most livestock have large rounded upper bodies and relatively slender limbs. The tamer is designed to restrain the body of the ungulate, leaving their limbs free. Most tamers are designed so the floor of the device will 'drop out' when the animal is positioned properly. Hoof care can be managed easily with an animal restrained in a tamer. The potential for injury is reduced because the limbs are unable to reach the ground.

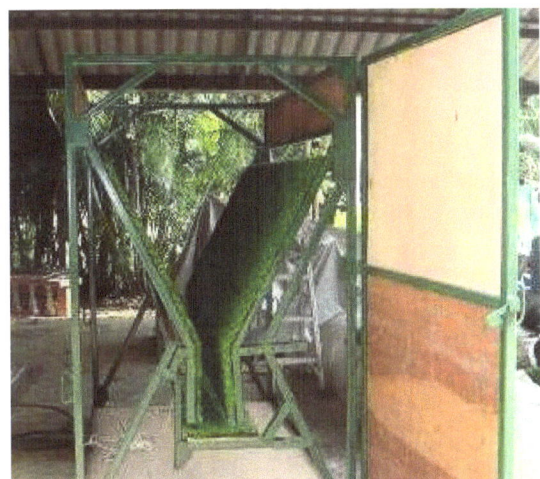

Figure 15: Tamer or drop chute (image from Deerfarmer.com)

Preventative Medicine

Herd management strategies are designed to optimize the success and health of the herd. Ultimately, the healthier the commodity the better the financial rewards. Livestock farmers will often treat the herd with medications and vaccines to afford the greatest protection from disease; the ramifications of not doing this may result in a catastrophic loss of animals and revenue. Individuals who may have a small number of animals may not treat them with all available preventative medicine products due to decreased risk and added costs.

Assortments of vaccines are available for ungulates; some are designed for specific species, while others, like Tetanus Toxoid, can be given to most types of ungulates.

Vaccine	Disease type	Symptoms
Scours	Viral, bacterial, protozoal	Diarrhea, dehydration
Clostridium	Bacterial	Variable depending on type
Foot Rot	Bacterial	Lameness, infected swollen feet
Leptospirosis	5 species of bacteria	Abortion, jaundice, hematuria
Mastitis	Bacterial	Swelling, infection
Pasteurella	Bacterial	Pneumonia
Pinkeye	Infectious, fly vectored	Conjunctivitis
Salmonella	Bacterial	Enteritis
Tetanus	Bacterial	Muscle rigidity
Vibriosis	Bacterial	Infertility, abortions

Table 10: Livestock vaccines

Deworming

As with horses and other species that feed off of the ground, parasitic infections can be common. For this reason, many species of livestock are placed on prophylactic dewormers. These products are very effective in eradicating ectoparasites and endoparasites, but tend not to afford much residual activity. Many livestock, therefore, receive deworming medication on a routine basis.

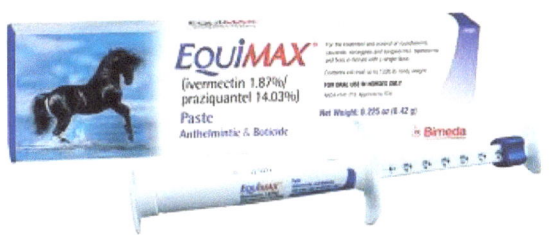

Figure 16: Livestock dewormer Ivermectin and Praziquantel

Product	Treatment
Doramectin	Ectoparasites
Moxidectin	Roundworms, lungworms, grubs, lice and mites
Ivermectin	Endoparasites and ectoparasites
Calf Pro	Coccidia
Deccox	Coccidia
Panacur	Roundworms, whipworms, hookworms, Taenia tapeworms
Praziquantel	Tapeworms, bots

Table 11: Antiparasitic medications

Hoof Care

The need for routine hoof care in livestock is based on several factors.

- Is there economic feasibility of maintaining hoof care?
- Are the substrate conditions conducive to normal hoof wear?
- Will the animal be processed prior to the need of hoof care?

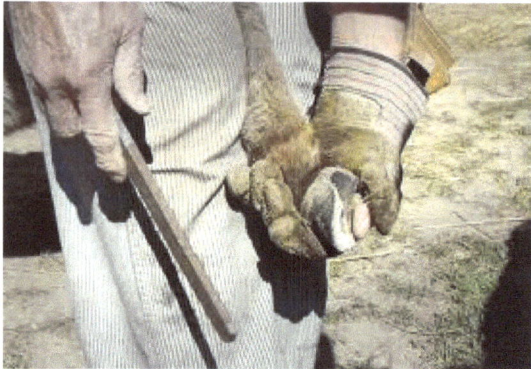

Figure 17: Clippers and files are used to trim and maintain ungulate hooves

Hoof trimming may require the use of a chute or chemical sedation to perform the procedure. Specialists called farriers are often needed to perform proper hoof trimming on ungulates.

Reproduction

Because livestock are valued as a commodity, reproduction and perpetuation of individuals is a necessity and can be profitable. The general reproductive strategy for ungulates is that in which a single dominant male oversees and breeds with a group of females. In this strategy, the male is the fittest and must defend that status from other males. The females benefit by breeding with the strongest individual and therefore ensuring their offspring are fit. Additionally, the females benefit from the protection the male provides. Like most animals, livestock have reproductively receptive seasons, and groups will often cycle at the same time. This means the male will often breed all of the individuals in the herd during this time, leading to synchronized parturition by the females.

Overall, livestock, and ungulates as a group, are effective producers of young. Once in labor, delivery is relatively quick, and dystocia is uncommon. Neonates are usually mobile shortly after delivery; most deliveries take place at night or in the twilight of the morning. Besides dystocia, other possible complications to labor include uterine prolapse and retained placenta. Uterine prolapse occurs when the act of labor causes the body of the uterus to invert itself and protrude from the vaginal vault. Retained placentas are a result of adhesions to the uterine wall that aren't broken down under normal circumstances. These reproductive complications can be managed medically, but given the nature of herd management of livestock, many are culled.

Care of the Neonate

Livestock and other ungulates rarely have problems associated with birthing and neonate care. Single births are most common, while twinning is rare. Ungulates will often give birth early in the morning; in the wild this strategy improves the chances of survival of both the neonate and the mother. Baby ungulates, once born, are able to stand and ambulate in a very short time; this too is a survival strategy found in the wild. Nursing occurs shortly after birth and continues multiple times daily for several weeks. Under normal conditions, neonates will develop rapidly, thriving on both its mother's milk and protection.

Occasionally a mother may not care for its neonate. Reasons for this may include:

- A sick or abnormal neonate. Neglect or abandonment in this case is a survival strategy seen in the wild.
- A first time mother unfamiliar with the duties of neonate care.
- An unhealthy mother unable to perform the duties of neonate care.

Usually in these cases, veterinary intervention is necessary to ensure the survival of the neonate. In most cases, intervention is in the form of bottle feeding of the neonate; this is sometimes referred to as 'hand-rearing' or 'assisted care'. Bottle feeding a receptive neonate can be very easy and rewarding; attempting to feed an unreceptive kid can be frustrating and lead to more invasive intervention such as intravenous nutrition. Several considerations must be made when hand-rearing a neonate.

- Is the milk-type appropriate for species being fed?
- Appropriate nipple size?
- Frequency of feedings?
- Volume given at each feeding?
- Will imprinting occur?

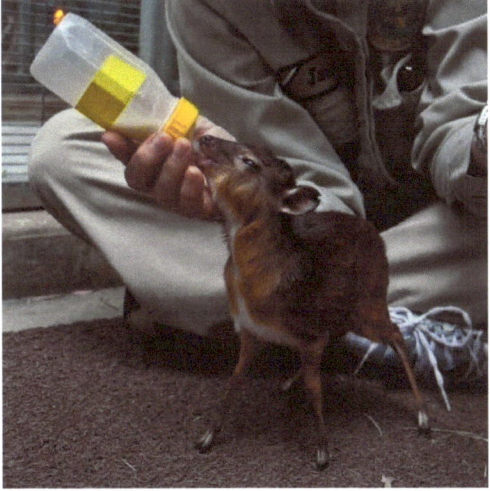

Figure 18: Baby ungulates are generally receptive to bottle feeding

Most of the information necessary for feeding a neonate is readily documented. Imprinting, however, is not often recognized until the neonate has become full grown and is no longer fearful of humans. This scenario can be very problematic for larger species of ungulates, as well as those with large pointy horns and antlers. Care must be used when considering and facilitating assisted care in these species.

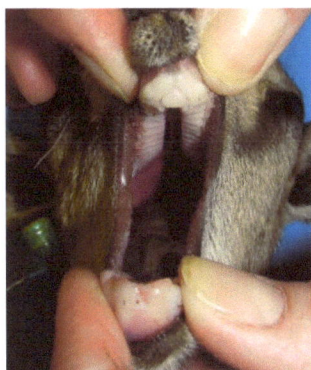

Figure 19: Cleft palate in a hoofstock

25

Species	Male	Female	Kid	Group
Cow	Bull	Cow	Calf	Herd
Sheep	Buck, Ram	Ewe, Dam	Lamb, Cosset	Flock, Herd
Goat	Buck, Billy	Doe, Nanny	Kid	Herd
Pig	Boar	Sow	Piglet, Shoat, Farrow	Herd, Sounder
Llama	Sire	Dam	Cria	Herd
Deer	Buck, Stag	Doe	Fawn	Herd

Table 12: Species names for various individuals

Diseases

A wide variety of diseases can affect livestock. The significance of this is compounded by the fact that livestock are often housed together or in close proximity. Transmission of disease in this type of setting can lead to increased mortality and morbidity of large numbers of individuals. Management of disease is often facilitated with vaccines, sanitary housing conditions, parasite control, high quality feeds and isolation or culling of diseased individuals.

Disease	Disease type	Susceptible Species	Treatment	Management
Anthrax	bacterial	cow, sheep, goat, pig, deer	antibiotics	vaccination
Brucellosis	bacterial	cow, sheep, goat, pig, deer	none	vaccination
BSE (mad cow disease)	prion	cow	none	cull
BVD (Bovine virus diarrhea)	virus	cow	none	vaccination, none
Calf Scours	bacteria, virus, protozoa	cow	antibiotics, fluid replacement	collostrum
Foot and Mouth	virus	cow, goat, sheep, pig, deer	none	slaughter, incineration
Foot Rot	bacterial	cow	antibiotics	prophylactic antibiotics and zinc
Johnes	bacterial	cow, sheep, goat, llama, deer	none	isolation, clean environment
Laminitis	inflammatory	horse, cow	mechanical support, analgesics	diet, early diagnosis
Scrapie	prion	sheep, goat	none	quarantine, slaughter
Tetanus	bacteria	horse, cow, sheep, goat, pig, deer	antibiotics	vaccination
Urolithiasis	mineral	cow, sheep, goat	adjust mineral intake, acidifiers	nutritional adjustment

Table 13: Diseases of livestock

Pocket Pets and Research Animals

Types

Pocket pets are usually thought of as small mammals, often rodents, which can fit in your pocket. Examples include mice, rats, hamsters, and sugar gliders, but also include much larger animals such as guinea pigs, rabbits, hedgehogs, chinchillas and ferrets. Most, with the exception of guinea pigs, rabbits and chinchillas are omnivorous. Pocket pets are used as a source of food, for pelts and in scientific research.

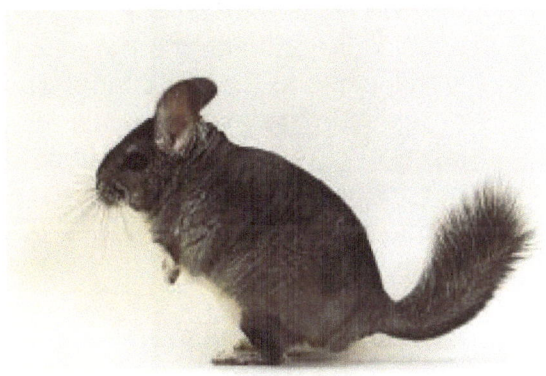

Figure 20: The Chinchilla is a rodent native to the Andes mountains of South America

Anatomy and Physiology

In general, the anatomy and physiology of pocket pets are not significantly different from that of companion animals. Because of the numbers of pocket pet species, it is often times easier to understand how their physiological parameters relate to other animals. Here are some assumptions to consider:

- Smaller mammals have higher metabolism.
- Smaller mammals have greater heat loss to body surface area ratios.
- Smaller mammals have higher heart rates and respiration rates to contend with higher metabolism and heat loss.
- Larger mammals have the opposite problems and typically have slower heart and respiration rates.
- Some animals are either crepuscular or nocturnal and may have different feeding and sleeping strategies.

Since most pocket pets are in the order Rodentia, their anatomy and physiology are characteristic of a herbivore. They can be further generalized as prey species. As mammals, this group would be characteristic of having reproduction, parturition and nursing common to placental species. Here are some additional generalizations about these animals to consider.

Coat

The hair-coat may be thick, soft, or in the case of hedgehogs, armadillos and porcupines, coarse, plated or quilled.
Fur color may be cryptic like wild counterparts or bred for unique color combinations.
Many species rely on self-grooming to maintain coat quality and typically do not require bathing.

Eyes

As a prey species, most pocket pets have side-oriented eye position.
Eyes may be large and have a tapetum lucitum to facilitate better vision at night.

Ears

Some pocket pets have large or delicate and vascular pinnas. Some get ectoparasites such as ear mites in their auditory canals.

Dentition

Rodents are characterized by having hypsodont dentition; teeth are constantly erupting and being worn down. Some may have brachydont dentition of the molars; teeth have a crown and root that does not erupt and wear down.

Central incisors are generally long and used for gnawing and cutting food such as plants and tubers. These teeth may require trimming.

Many rodents have yellow or brown teeth; this is considered normal coloration and can be due to iron pigments in the tooth enamel.

The oral cavity is generally small and difficult to visualize.

Feet

Feet may be used for digging or foraging; nails may be long and sharp and may require periodic trimming.

Digestion

The basic digestive system of the herbivore consists of a stomach, small and large intestine and a well developed cecum. The intestines are longer than a carnivore because plant material requires more 'digestive time'. Feces are commonly pelleted.

Reproduction

Reproductive anatomy may be difficult to visualize. The penis may be retractable in many species, and the scrotum may be small, close to the abdominal wall or reside in the abdomen.

Many pocket pets have multiple offspring often called a 'litter'. Many pocket pets are born without fur and are initially unable to see.

Most can procreate frequently producing several litters each year.

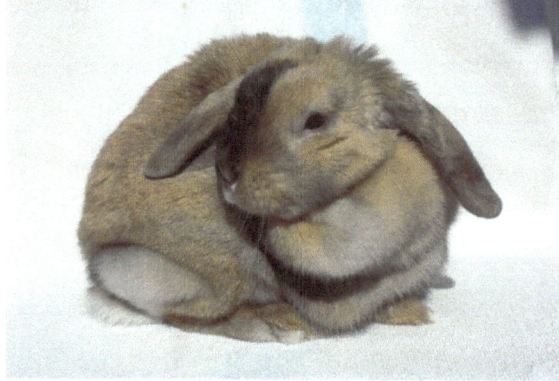

Figure 21: Lagomorphs include rabbits, hares and pikas; the domestic rabbit includes nearly fifty breeds recognized by the American Rabbit Breeders Association.

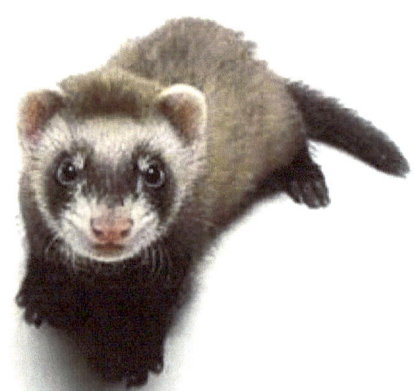

Figure 22: Ferrets, also called pole cats, are carnivorous predators belonging to the family Mustelidae and are related to the endangered Black-footed Ferret.

Species	Longevity (years)	Gestation (days)	Litter size	Special concerns	Diet	Copro-phagia
Mouse	1-3	19-21	7-12	Skin of tail can be 'degloved' if pulled Red tears Cedar/pine respiratory problems	Omnivorous; pellet, seeds, berries, bugs	no
Rat	2-4	21-23	8-12	Cedar and pine bedding is toxic to rats. Red tears-red discharge from eyes called porphyrin	Omnivorous	no
Hamster	2-3	15-18	4-12	Antisocial, tend to bite	pellet, vegetables and fruit	yes
Guinea Pig	5-7	63	1-6	Precocial kits	Pellet, vegetables, hay, fruit	yes
Chinchilla	15-20	111	2-6	Dust bath weekly	Roughage, pellets	yes
Rabbit	4-8	28-31	2-6	Easily fracture back	Pellet, vegetables and fruit	yes
Ferret	5-8	42	10	Females regulated/illegal in some states	Obligate carnivores	no

Table 14: Pocket pet vital statistics

Physical Exam

Overall, the physical exam of a pocket pet should proceed in the same manner as any companion animal. By maintaining consistency with the physical exam process, no matter what the species, the thoroughness of the exam will be maintained. Some aspects of the exam, however, may need to be adjusted based on patient size or morphology. Here are some general considerations and recommendations:

- Examine the patient from cranial to caudal. This enables you to greet the patient and see its temperament.
- After examination of the patient's head, cover it with a towel; this may have a calming effect on the patient.
- The heart and respiration rates may be rapid. Count the number of heartbeats and breaths in a ten second period and multiply those numbers by six to get the rates per minute.
- Use a stethoscope with a small pediatric bell to hear the heart more accurately.
- Use care when inserting a rectal thermometer as tissues are delicate in this area.

29

Restraint

Proper restraint is essential for safe and effective patient examination and manipulation. The primary weapon of pocket pets is their sharp teeth that can deliver a significant bite. Proper restraint of the head as well as the use of protective equipment such as gloves is essential. Some pocket pets can be restrained by the 'scruff' effectively eliminating their ability to bite.

Some species such as armadillos and hedgehogs are able to roll-up into a ball as a means of defense, making them difficult to manipulate. These animals may need to be anesthetized in order to properly restrain and examine them. Placing these animals on a clear Plexiglas surface will often allow for visualization of their underside when they 'unroll'.

Injection Sites

The methods and locations of injections in pocket pets are very similar to those of companion animals; the most significant difference is patient size. Necessary adjustments when giving injections to pocket pets include the use of smaller gauge needles and careful attention to injection techniques to insure proper placement of medications. Additionally, some species have very thin and delicate skin; care must be taken not to eviscerate the skin with the needle or tear the skin with overly aggressive restraint.

Injection Type	AKA	Injection Angle	Locations	Comments
Subcutaneous	SQ,SC	45°	Interscapular (IS)	Can be given in other areas where the skin can be tented.
Intramuscular	IM	90°	Muscles of the limbs	Avoid the sciatic nerve in the rear limbs.
Intravenous	IV	15-30°	Jugular, Cephalic, Saphenous, Femoral, Vena cava	In very small species, the femoral vein may be the only option; sampling from the vena cava should only be done by experienced individuals.

Note: Always aspirate syringe prior to injecting, there should be no air or blood.

Table 15: Injection types and sites for pocket pets

Preventative Medicine

Preventative health care for pocket pets, although an important consideration, tends to be less utilized than those for companion animals such as dogs and cats. Some people may be reluctant to spend fifty dollars each year for a veterinary exam on a five dollar hamster. Luckily for hamsters and other pocket pets, they tend to be self-maintaining when given a proper diet and housing.

Types of preventative medicine available to pocket pets may include:

- Routine physical exam
- Deworming or antiparasitic treatment
- Teeth and nail trimming
- Bathing and grooming
- Vaccinations
- Spay and neuter

The most common of the above procedures includes spaying, neutering and teeth and nail trimming. Spaying and neutering insure that offspring are not produced. Many people desire a pair of rabbits and not a menagerie. In some species such as ferrets, spaying and neutering causes a reduction of musk scent production.

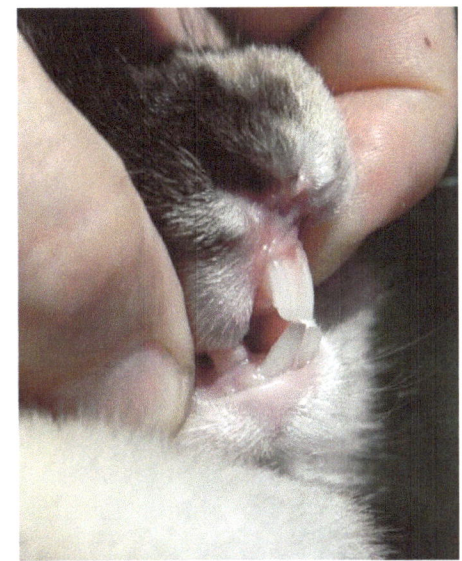

Figure 24: Normal rabbit incisors. Rabbits have four incisors on the upper arcade, two behind the outer primary set.

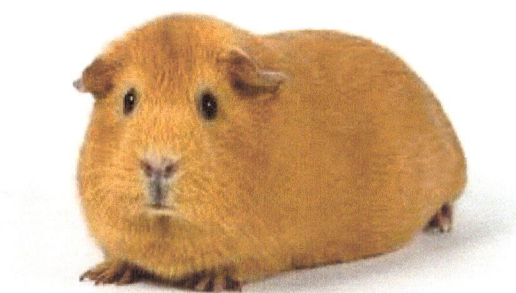

Figure 23: The Guinea Pig or Cavy, is native to South America. There are thirteen breeds of domestic cavies.

Species	Disease	Symptoms	Treatment
Mouse	Obesity Neoplasia CMP (chronic murine pneumonia) Mycoplasma	Masses Upper respiratory symptoms Respiratory symptoms/discharge	Surgical removal Antibiotics Antibiotics, proper nutrition
Rat	Obesity Rat bite fever	Bacterial disease	Carriers, zoonotic
Hamster	Wet tail	Diarrhea, lethargy	
Guinea Pig	Scurvy Parasites	Lethargy, weight loss Diarrhea	Vitamin C Antiparasitic medications
Chinchilla	Enteritis Respiratory disease	Diarrhea, abdo pain Eye/nose discharge	Generally fatal Supportive care
Rabbit	Snuffles(pasteurellosis) Bordetella	Sneezing, nasal discharge Eye/nose discharge, pneumonia	No treatment Antibiotics
Ferret	Hyperadrenal (Addisons) disease Insulinomas	Hair loss, pruritis Lethargy, hypoglycemia	Surgical removal of adrenal gland Steroids, removal of pancreatic tumor

Table 16: Common diseases of pocket pets

Anesthesia

Pocket pets can be easily induced and maintained under anesthesia with gas anesthetics such as isoflurane. Animals can be masked under manual restraint or an induction chamber can be used. Injectable anesthetic drugs may be used in larger animals such as rabbits. Anesthetic 'cocktails' such as ketamine and xylazine can be injected easily, but may increase recovery time when compared to inhalant anesthetics. Most pocket pets are not intubated because they are too small or difficult to do so. A 'blind intubation' can be performed on rabbits; with the rabbit in an upright position, the endotracheal tube is advanced down the throat. Respiratory sounds are listened for while advancing the tube into the trachea.

Nutrition

Most pocket pets are fed manufactured diets that are formulated and nutritionally balanced. These feeds are usually in the form of extruded pellets and are generally sized to the specific needs of the animal. In some cases, however, large biscuits are made and the animal chews the corners of the food item rather than ingesting a whole pellet.

Natural food items such as Timothy hay, vegetables and fruits may be given to further balance or enhance the diet of these species. Guinea pigs require vitamin C in their diet, and supplementing them with oranges can facilitate that dietary need.

Moderation is paramount to any feeding strategy. Too much fruits and vegetables can lead to diarrhea; whereas, a lack of them may cause other digestion problems. Feeds should be rationed out appropriately in order to reduce the incidence of obesity in these animals.

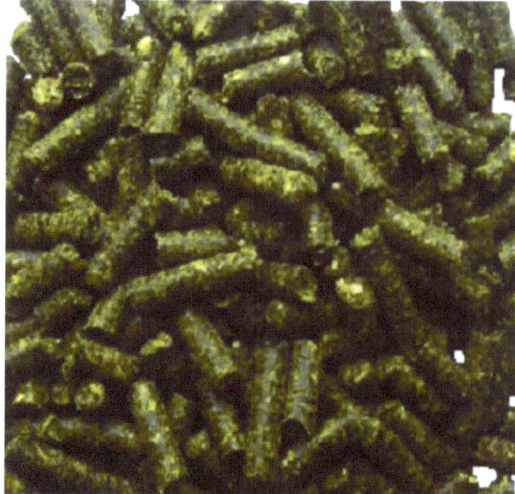

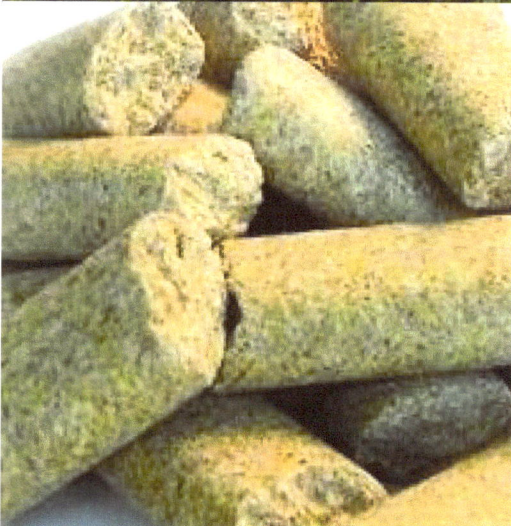

Figure 25: Rabbit pellets (top) and rodent chow (bottom) shown in actual proportions

Some pocket pets will eat their feces to improve digestion or help maintain adequate bacterial flora. The process, called coprophagia, is an important facet of rabbit, hamster, chinchilla and guinea pig digestion.

Water should be available at all times, and lick drinkers are very affective at delivering water without waste or evaporation. A ball bearing at the end of the drinking tube serves to prevent dripping, but allows water to pass when dislodged by the act of drinking or licking. Water bottles should be cleaned and changed regularly in order to prevent algae buildup.

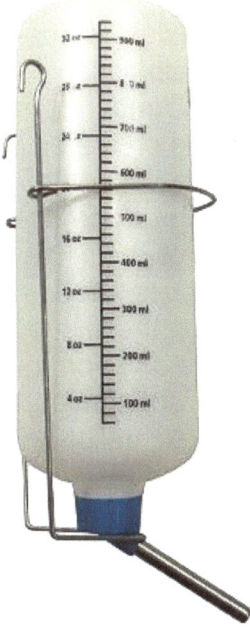

Figure 26: Commonly used pocket pet drinker

Hand raising rodents can be challenging and rewarding. Rehabilitation facilities deal with orphaned neonate wildlife such as rabbits, squirrels, opossums and skunks. Orphaned wildlife, especially rabbits, can be difficult to hand raise due to the special dietary needs and fragility of these altricial species. Just as milk replacement products made for dogs and cats, some manufacturers offer milk replacers for exotics.

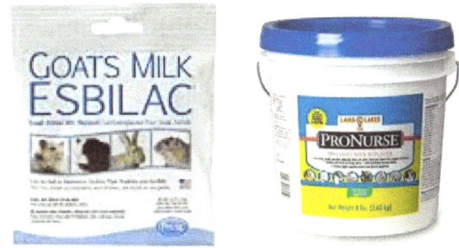

Figure 27: Milk replacement products for pocket pets and other exotic animals

Reproduction

Pocket pets are prolific breeders. Many species are rodents and generally have large litters. Most rodent pocket pets, with the exception of guinea pigs and chinchillas, have altricial babies. Altricial, meaning to require nourishment, is depicted by hairless babies with closed eyes. These babies are completely dependent on their parents until their eyes open and they further develop. Both altricial and precocial species will nurse mother's milk until they have transitioned to a solid diet. The time at which this occurs is called weaning. Once weaned, the offspring are generally independent and can be separated. In some cases, the mother may already be pregnant and near delivery when the first offspring are weaned.

Reproduction can be triggered by a multitude of things in species that spontaneously ovulate. Estrus and pheromones will stimulate individuals to breed; the introduction of new individuals may have a similar effect. Gender dynamics can be a factor in reproduction and reproductive success. Most rodents like mice and rats, will be better situated for breeding when two or more females are set-up with a single male. Additionally, the females should be placed in the male's cage, and not vice versa. Having more than one male in a breeding situation can lead to aggression and fighting between males; this ultimately leads to low productivity. Once bred, most females are separated from the male, as his role in nurturing the offspring is minimal.

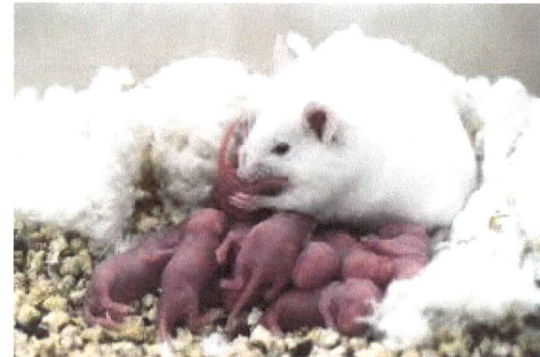
Figure 28: Female white mouse and her litter of pups

Reproductive Anatomy

Many pocket pets are small and difficult to ascertain gender. Some have external genitalia, while others only have small protrusions. Some, like mice and rats, have the ability to retract their testicles, so they may or may not be visible. Anal-genital distance may be used in most species to determine gender; the distance in females may be nearly half that of males.

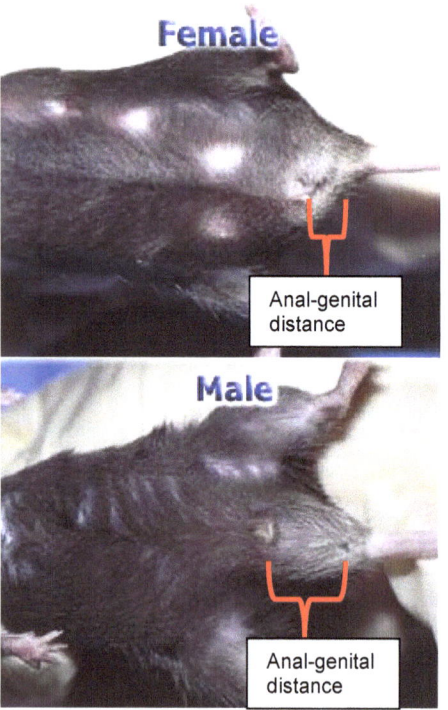

Female

Anal-genital distance

Male

Anal-genital distance

Figure 29: Gender determination in the mouse (ALAAS learning library)

Adult male rabbits have scrotal sacks that can be easily visualized; this may be more challenging in young male rabbits.

The penis in many species can be extruded by digital manipulation. With the animal in dorsal recumbency, digital pressure can be placed on the proximal aspect of the genital opening. If male, the penis will begin to protrude with slight pressure. If female, some tissue will protrude, but its appearance is not phallus-like. In females, the tissue appears more concave and somewhat vulva-like. Do not over-manipulate the genitalia, as this tissue is delicate and can be injured if not careful.

Research

Scientific research is an important aspect of human medicine. Annually, scientific research is a multi-billion dollar endeavor. The use of animals to test new medications or to learn about disease processes has been going on for hundreds of years. The genetic types of animals used are very specific and breeding particular genetic lines is equally important. Mice and rats are considered good scientific models due to their rapid maturation and prolific breeding. The rabbit, guinea pig, hamster and gerbil are used by the research community. Zebra fish are popular in research because of the following rationale:

- Embryos are transparent allowing the visualization of all developmental stages with great clarity.
- Embryonic development is rapid, and all common vertebrate specific body features can be seen within two days of development

- The genome of Zebra fish is sequenced
- Short generation time (2-4 months)
- Drugs can be administered directly to fish water or by microinjection
- Ease in handling and inexpensive in comparison to other vertebrate research models

All research animals are protected by the Animal Welfare Act (AWA), and all research facilities are inspected regularly. The institutional animal care and use committee (IACUC) oversees all experimentation and research practices on all animals used in science. Violations in animal care and well being can lead to the termination of an experiment, costing the researcher both time and money.

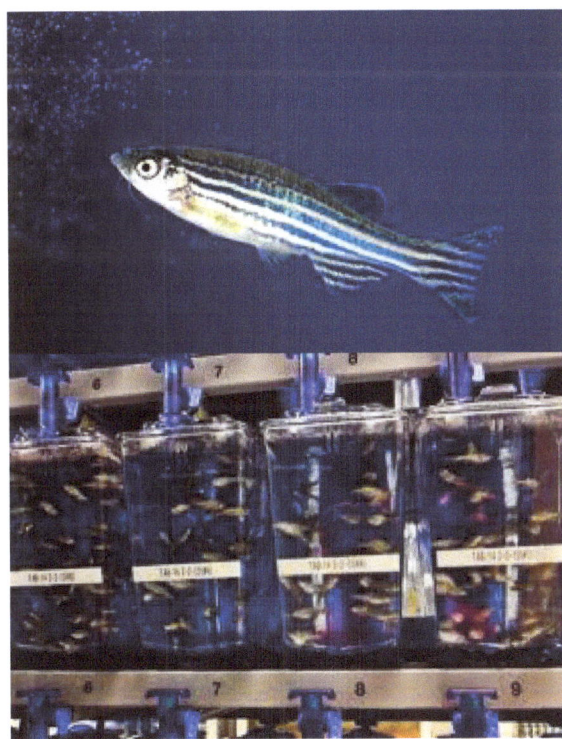

Figure 30: Zebra fish (top) are becoming increasingly popular for scientific research. They can be housed in small tanks with filtration systems (bottom)

Animals used for research are provided with necessities for proper health and nutrition, and in some species, provided with enrichment. Items used for enrichment may include boomer balls, metal chains or even PVC pipe fittings. The documentation process for animal use is rigorous, and in most cases, funding or approval is not obtained. In the few cases that go to experimentation, the process may be long; most new drugs or treatments take ten to fifteen years to get to the consumer.

Housing

Most research animals, if large, are housed individually or in numbers dictated by the IUCUC. Rabbits may be housed separately; whereas, mice and rats may be housed in groups. Rabbits are housed in traditional wire cages, however, rats and mice tend to be contained in plastic boxes. These boxes contain food and water, and in some cases, are connected to a ventilation system to remove ammonia urine smells from the air.

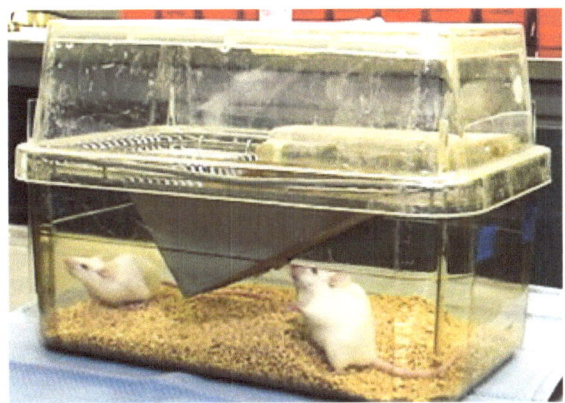

Figure 31: Research mouse box (AALAS learning library)

Substrates may be wood shavings or cellulose, all of which absorb urine and moisture from water sources. Bedding is usually changed weekly, along with food and water. Some animals may be involved with diabetes testing and require frequent bedding changes due to increased water consumption and urination associated with that disease.

Management

The ultimate goal of research is to demonstrate efficacy of a drug or technique; the animal model is the step before clinical human trials. If effective, the end results are drugs and procedures that can save and treat human medical diseases. Most research studies are terminal for the animal; their contribution is the understanding of scientific queries. Once all the information is gleaned from the animals, euthanasia is performed. In small pocket pets like mice and rats, euthanasia is performed using carbon dioxide (CO_2) gas. In high concentrations, CO_2 gas displaces oxygen and causes asphyxiation. The animals initially go to sleep; this is quickly followed by death. A secondary form of euthanasia is performed after the CO_2 administration. In mice, cervical dislocation is an acceptable secondary technique for confirming death, while in rats, a bilateral thoracotomy is performed. In other species, including rabbits and guinea pigs, euthanasia is performed with an intravenous overdose of pentobarbital. Death in these species can be confirmed with cardiac auscultation.

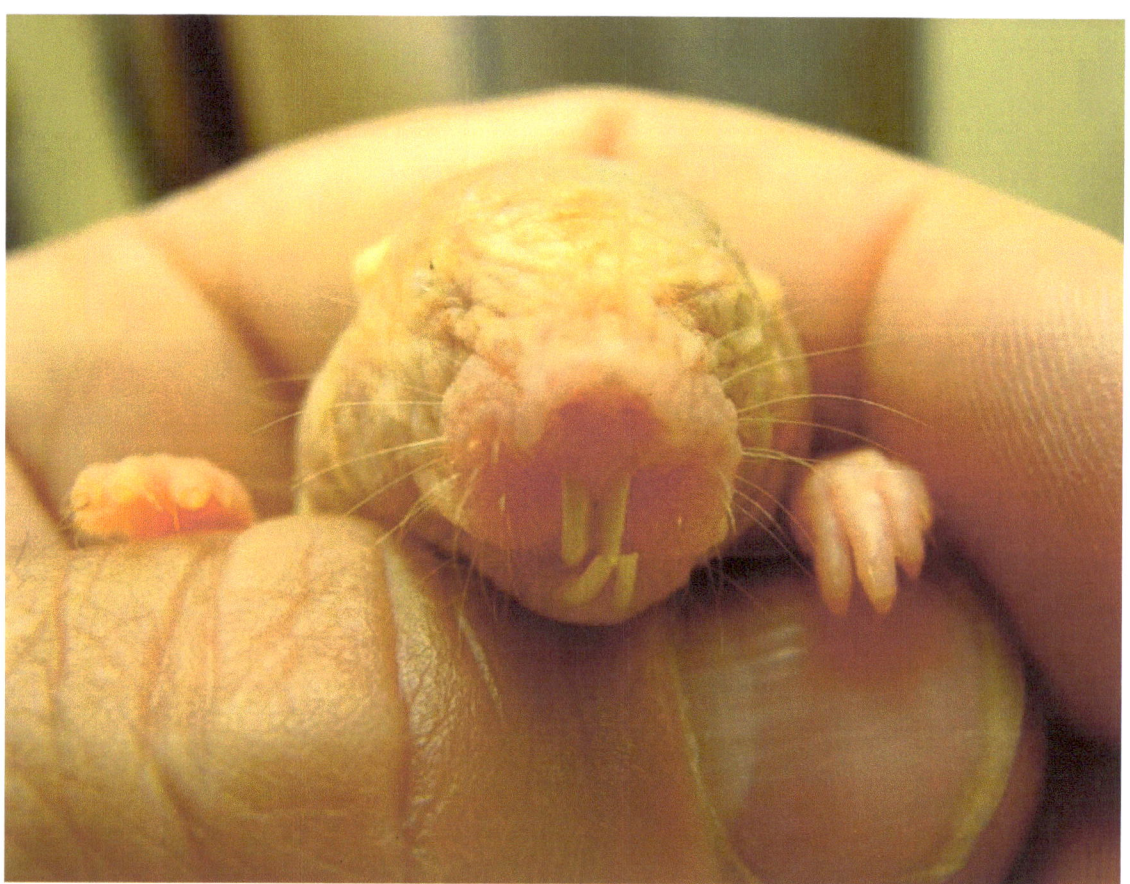

Figure 32: The Naked Mole-rat is unique in the rodent family in that they are surprisingly long lived when compared to their mice and rat cousins. Naked Mole-rats have been known to live over thirty years in captivity.

Zoo Animals

Zoos are home to the most diverse collection of exotic animals outside of the wild. Any wild animal, no matter if captive bred, imprinted or habituated, has the potential to exhibit wild behaviors including aggression. For this reason, nearly all exotic zoo animals are anesthetized for handling or medical procedures. Additionally, husbandry practices include protective measures that limit or preclude contact with these animals no matter how docile or tractable. Most dangerous animals such as large carnivores, have an exhibit area as well as an off exhibit bedroom area where they can be held during exhibit maintenance and cleaning.

Zoo Medicine

Zoo veterinary care and preventative medicine are no different from other veterinary fields. The client, however, is the zoological institution and animal keeper, and decisions about medical care are made by animal curators, managers and veterinarians. Factors that are considered when attempting medical care on zoo animals include feasibility of medical care, likelihood of medical success, and the importance of the animal in conservation efforts. For example, an ungulate with good genetic representation and a leg fracture may not receive surgical repair due to its less significant value and difficulty in managing this type of medical problem. In these cases, the animals may be euthanized. In other cases, heroic measures may be taken to manage medical ailments. Anesthesia is a necessity in most cases, and needs to be considered when managing cases where long term nursing care is needed.

Other factors, such as reintroduction dynamics and species importance are considered when choosing to hospitalize an exotic animal.

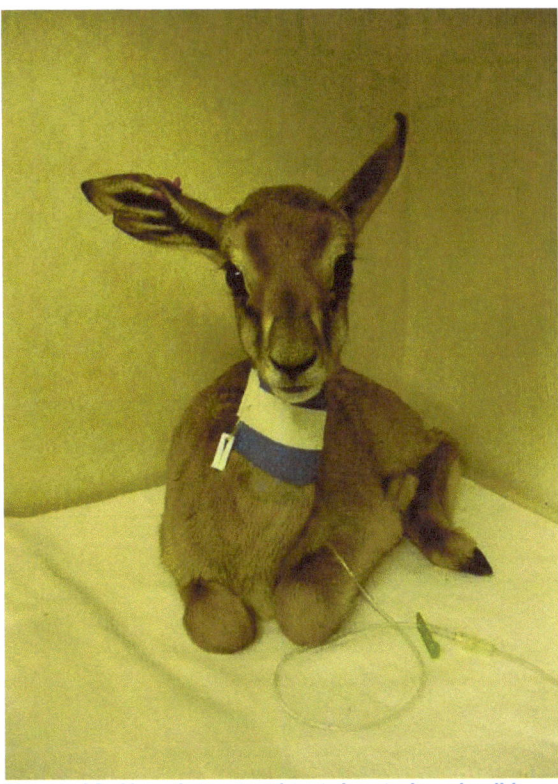

Figure 33: Ungulates tend to tolerate jugular IV catheters

Sick ungulates are generally tolerant of intravenous catheters and fluid administration, however, carnivores and primates may be more likely to chew or remove bandaging and catheters once placed. Some species requiring intravenous fluids may need to receive a constant rate infusion (CRI) of an anesthetic/analgesic such as ketamine in order to manage them safely. Primates with IV catheters placed in their posterior saphenous veins may benefit with having their whole leg bandaged and immobilized so they cannot manipulate the catheter site.

37

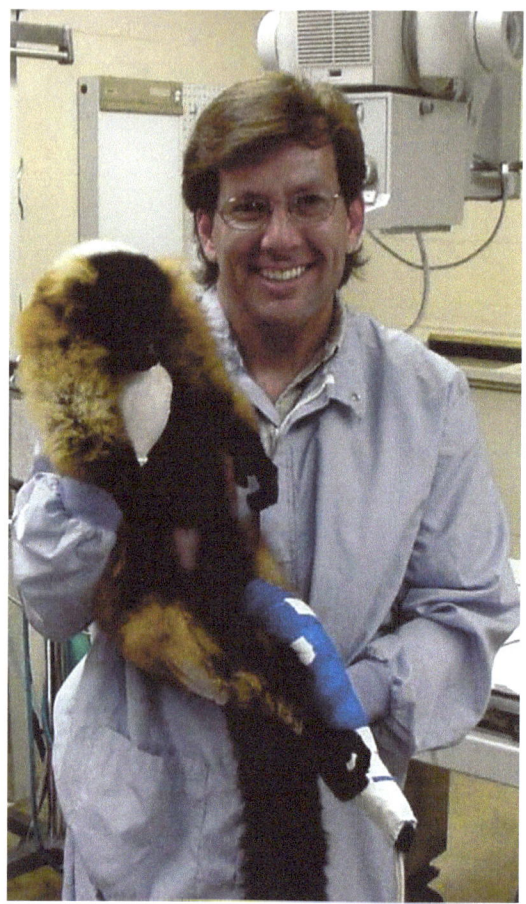

Figure 34: The author holding a Red-ruffed Lemur with an IV catheter and bandage on the left leg

Anatomical and physiological anomalies are present in zoo species, but most are similar to a particular domestic species; a zebra is like a horse, tiger is like a domestic cat, a hyena is like a domestic dog, and so on.

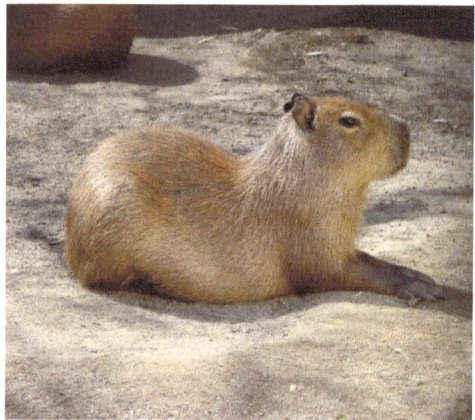

Figure 35: The Capybara, the world's largest rodent, is similar in appearance to a domestic guinea pig

When working with exotic and zoo animals, human safety is paramount. The standard protocol for any dangerous animal escape is to use deadly force in order to protect public safety. That being said, cages, doors, crates and exhibits that house dangerous animals have been designed for the utmost protection and safety so the animal is protected from being placed in a lethal situation.

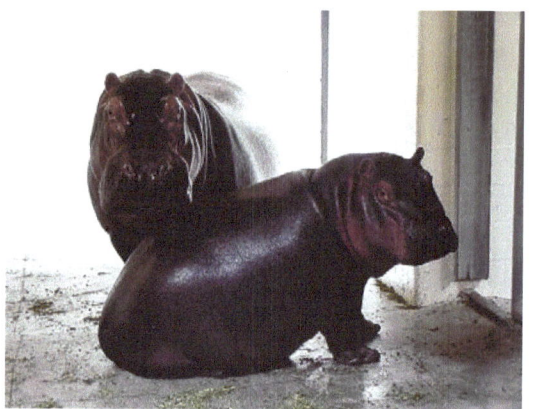

Figure 36: Hippo's are one of the most dangerous animals in Africa

The Zoo Veterinary Practice

A zoo veterinary practice is set up much like a small animal practice, with diagnostic equipment such as radiography and ultrasound, treatment, ICU and surgical facilities as well as holding facilities for hospitalized patients. There are generally one or more veterinarians, veterinary technicians and hospital keepers. Additionally, diagnostic laboratory staff may be employed to process samples obtained during medical procedures. Most zoos lack the resources to maintain equipment such as CT and MRI machines; frequently these modalities are provided by local veterinary specialty facilities or human medical hospitals.

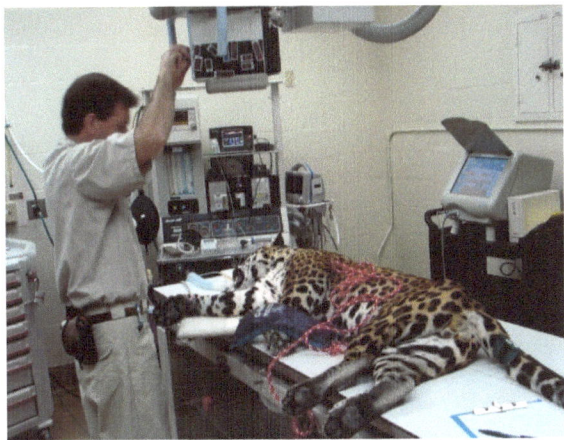

Figure 37: Radiology is commonly used in zoo veterinary practices; here, the author takes radiographs of a jaguar

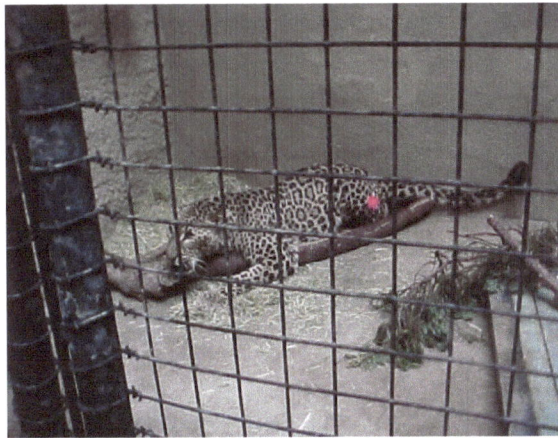

Figure 38: A jaguar after being injected with a remote injection system or dart.

Anesthesia

Safe handling of dangerous zoo animal species requires anesthesia in most cases. Even non-dangerous species such as birds and non-venomous reptiles benefit from the use of anesthetics for medical procedures. For example, survey radiographs (two views) of a bird can be undertaken in less than ten minutes with anesthesia; the same procedure may take longer with more potential injury to the bird when anesthesia is not used. For birds, anesthesia can be induced and maintained with a facemask; whereas, most large birds and mammals may require injectable anesthetics. Injectable anesthetics for zoo animals are usually delivered in the following manner:

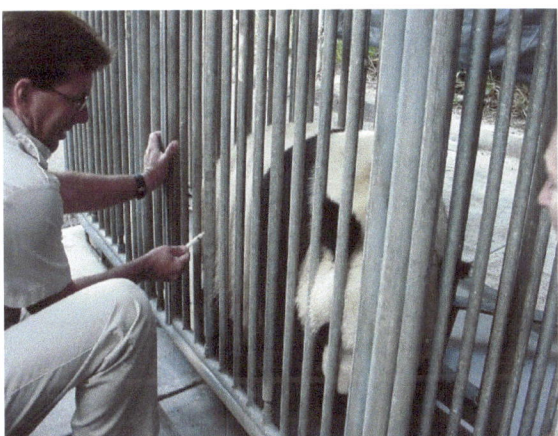

Figure 39: The author giving a vaccine to a Giant Panda using a squeeze cage; note the back side of the cage is 'squeezed' towards the front side enabling the injection.

- Using manual restraint with a net, gloves or push board
- Using behavioral restraint by stationing the animal for hand injection
- Using squeezing devises in which one wall can be closed in on the animal causing them to 'squeeze ' against the cage bars
- Using remote injection systems to deliver injectable drugs from afar.

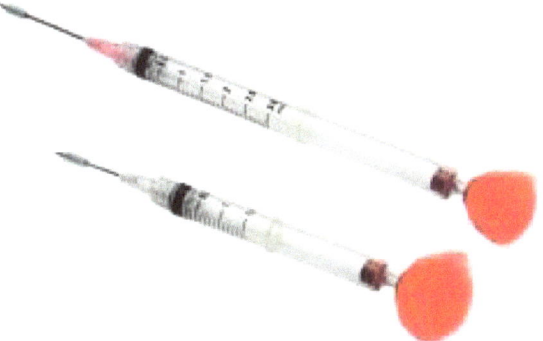

Figure 40: Remote injection systems utilize a syringe dart that is delivered by an air driven pistol or rifle.

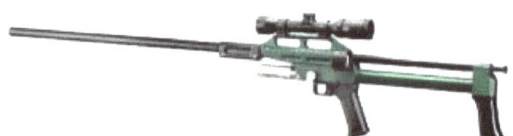

Figure 41: A typical remote injection dart rifle. Rifles, with longer barrel lengths than pistols, tend to be more accurate at longer distances.

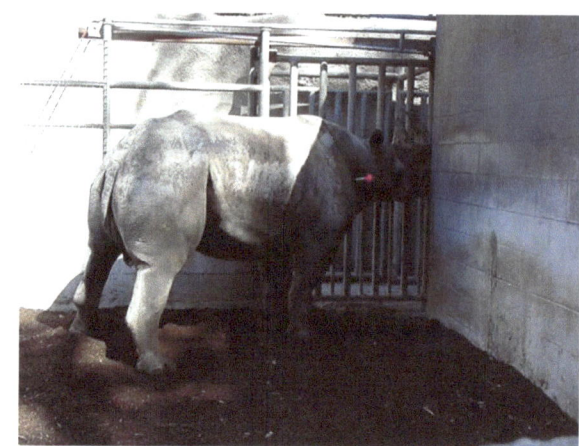

Figure 43: A black Rhinoceros demonstrating a narcotic 'head push' prior to anesthetic collapse.

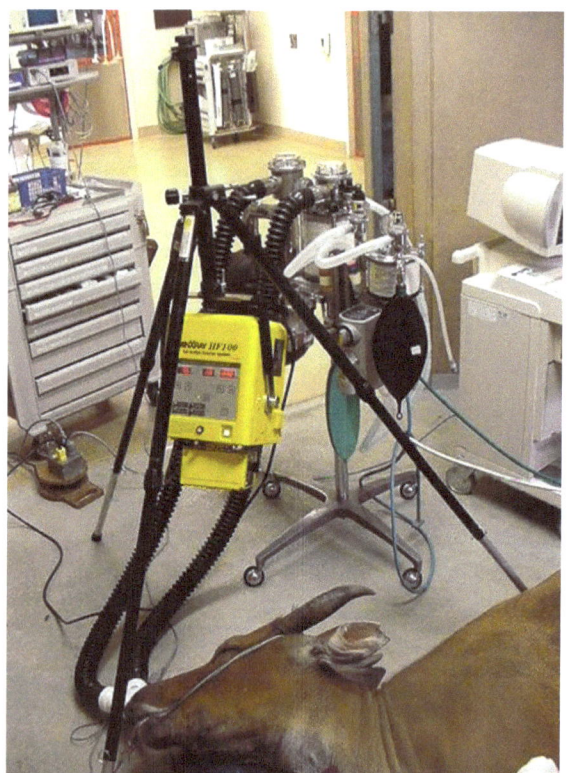

Figure 42: Large animals may require the use of the floor instead of a surgical table.

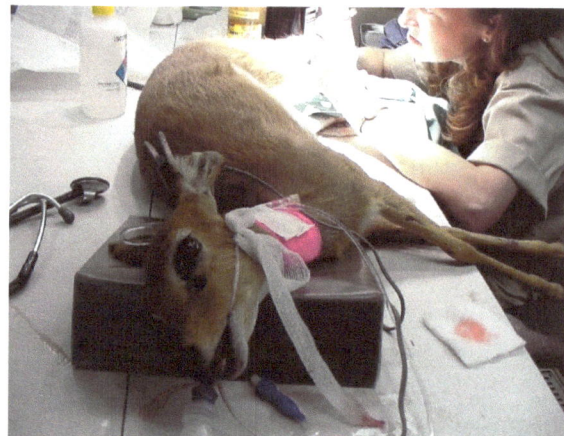

Figure 44: Elevating the head with the mouth pointed down is a safe position for ruminants; this allows saliva and potential regurgitation to drain out from the oral cavity.

The use of potent narcotics such as carfentanil and ectorphine has allowed zoo veterinarians to immobilize large and dangerous animals quickly and safely. These potent opiod based narcotics cause fast induction of anesthesia, and rapid recovery with the use of reversing agents also known as antagonists..

Medication Administration

Zoo animals can be notoriously difficult to medicate. Distasteful medications and the restraint necessary to facilitate medicating some animals, has lead to creative strategies for medication administration. Hiding medications in food items has long been a strategic means of medication administration. Compounded medications can also be used to reduce the potent taste of some medications. When all else fails, injectable medications can be given, making note of where the injection was given in order to repeat subsequent injections in that area. Birds are often gavaged medications in order to ensure medication compliance. Medications placed on food or in water can be variable in their compliance, especially in multi-individual exhibits. At times medicated food and water have been used to prophylactially treat an exhibit of conspecific individuals.

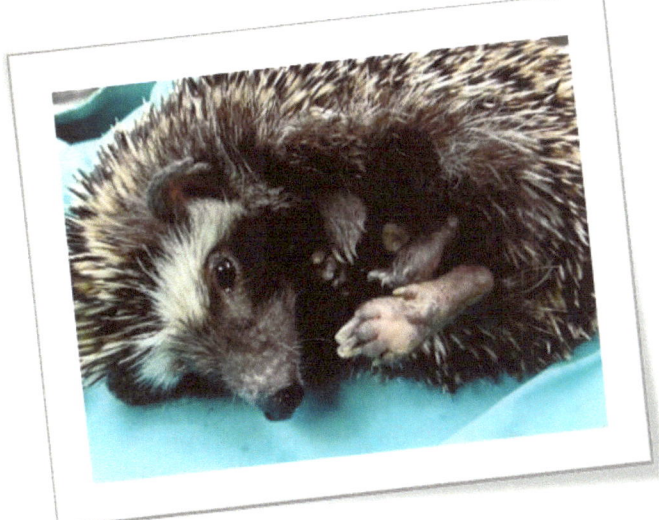

African Hedgehog

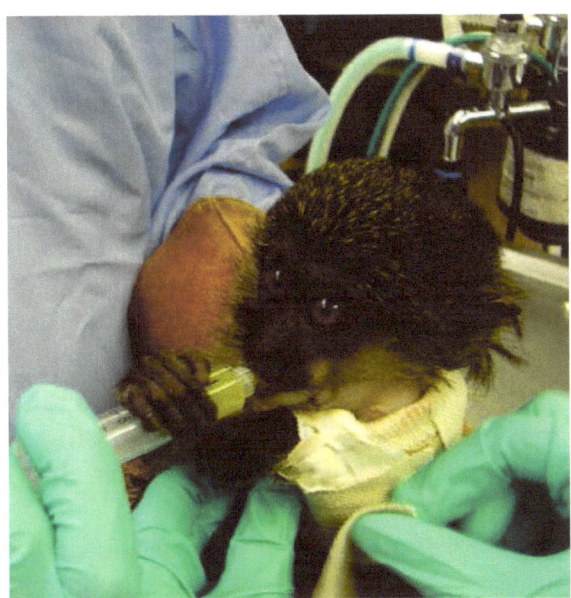

Figure 45: Allens Swamp Monkey receiving oral medication

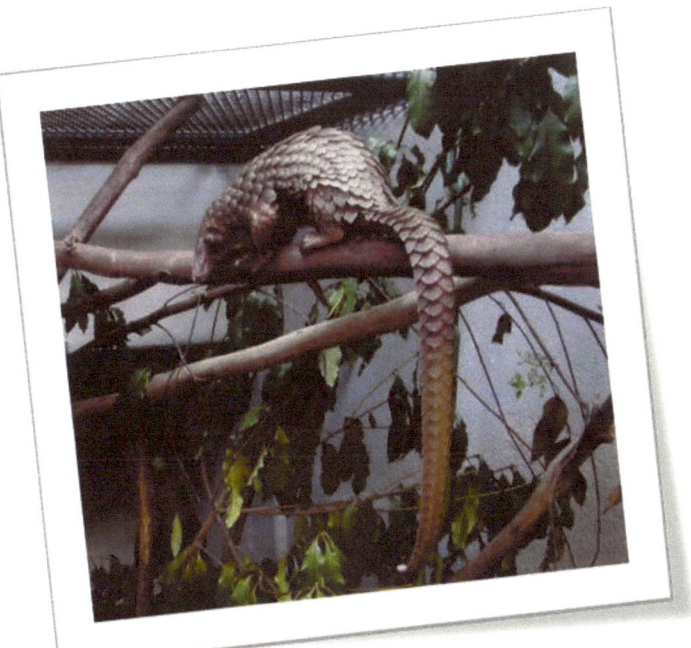

Tree Pangolin

Bird Medicine

Birds are a highly specialized group of animals. Most of the nearly ten thousand species of birds are characterized by having feathers and being capable of flight; whereas, over forty species of terrestrial birds including emus, ostriches, kiwis and penguins are considered flightless. All birds lay eggs. Taxonomically, birds reside in the class Aves, and include psittacines (parrots), passerines (sparrows et. al.) and falciformes (hawks and falcons), all of which are common companion species. Some birds are highly social and intelligent, while others can mimic human words and sounds in their vocalizations. Some species are used for hunting; the sport of falconry utilizes raptors to catch prey animals for sustenance. Cormorants were once used to catch fish; a tether was placed around the bird's neck to prevent it from swallowing the fish and flying away.

Birds eat a variety of foods including fruits, seeds, fish and flesh, while others drink nectar or as with flamingoes, sift krill. Living birds lack teeth, but many have sharp hooked or powerful beaks made of keratin; some show adaptations for probing for food, and others have specialized beaks for accessing specifically shaped flowers. Birds play an important role in insect control, flower pollination and seed dispersal.

Birds possess highly specialized scales called feathers; they function to provide flight for most birds in addition to protection and insulation from the environment. Feathers are also used during breeding and mate selection.

Most hummingbirds weigh as little as five grams, about the weight of a US nickel, while the largest bird, the ostrich, may weigh over one hundred and fifty kilograms. The heaviest flying birds, however, include the Mute Swan and African Kori Bustard, each weighing about twenty kilograms.

Modern birds originated from dinosaurs that, like archaeopteryx, had bird-like features including feathers. These predecessors had bony tails, teeth, wings, clawed fingers and were likely better gliders than fliers. The trend for more proficient flight caused the need for reduction in anatomical features to reduce weight. Structures such as the bony tail and teeth were lost, while the fusion of the ribcage and the development of a keel and furculum for powered flight were making birds better fliers. Reptilian features still exist in modern birds, most notably, their scaled legs and feet.

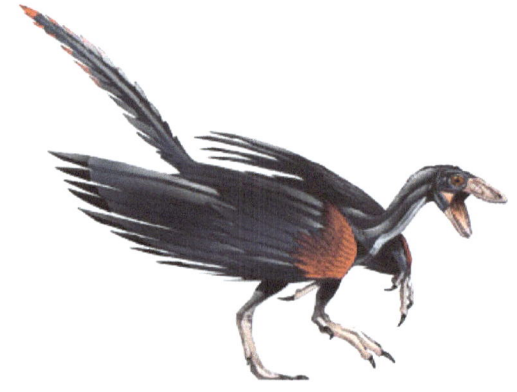

Figure 46: Archaeopteryx courtesy of Fossil.Wikia.com

42

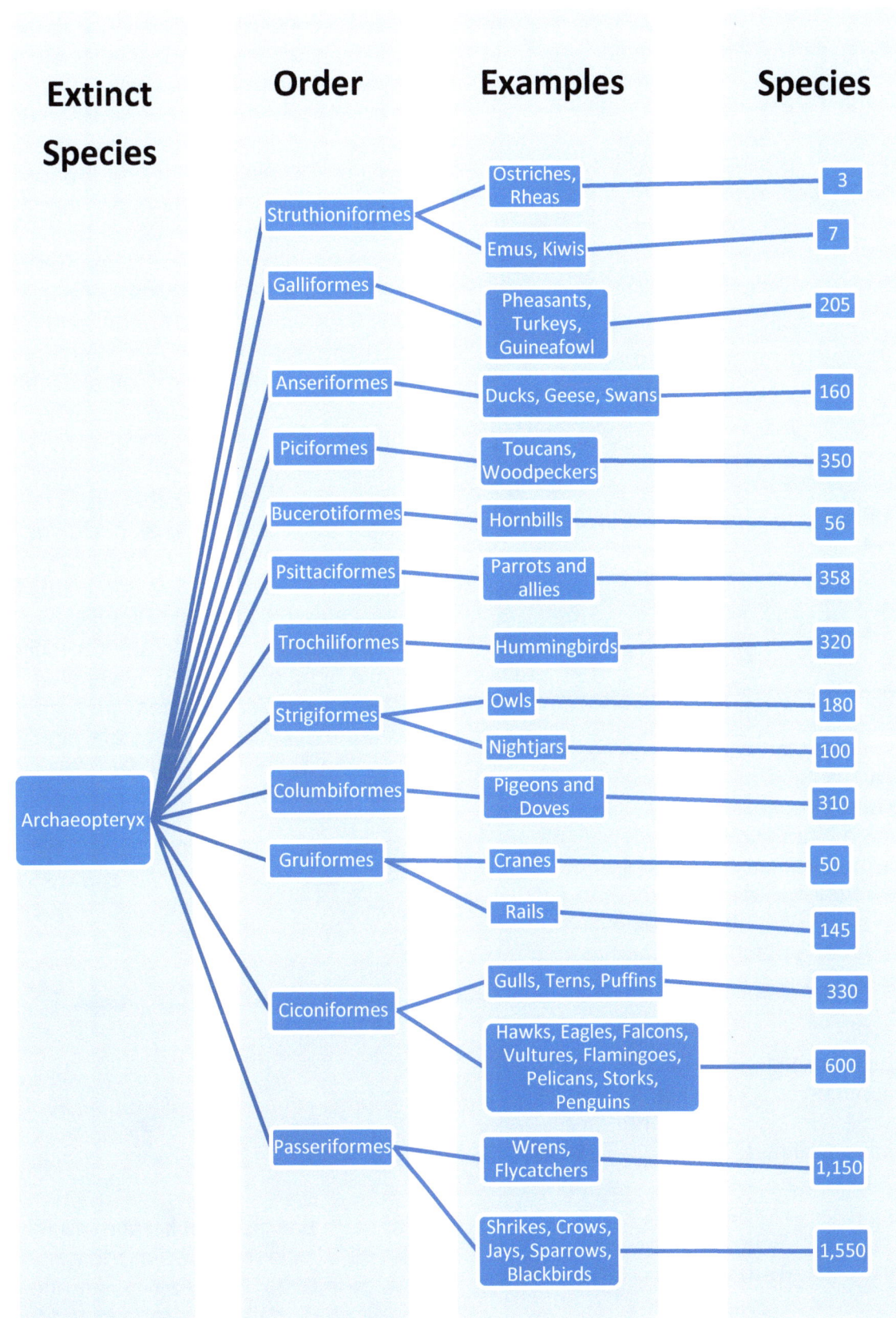

Extinct Species	Order	Examples	Species
Archaeopteryx	Struthioniformes	Ostriches, Rheas	3
		Emus, Kiwis	7
	Galliformes	Pheasants, Turkeys, Guineafowl	205
	Anseriformes	Ducks, Geese, Swans	160
	Piciformes	Toucans, Woodpeckers	350
	Bucerotiformes	Hornbills	56
	Psittaciformes	Parrots and allies	358
	Trochiliformes	Hummingbirds	320
	Strigiformes	Owls	180
		Nightjars	100
	Columbiformes	Pigeons and Doves	310
	Gruiformes	Cranes	50
		Rails	145
	Ciconiformes	Gulls, Terns, Puffins	330
		Hawks, Eagles, Falcons, Vultures, Flamingoes, Pelicans, Storks, Penguins	600
	Passeriformes	Wrens, Flycatchers	1,150
		Shrikes, Crows, Jays, Sparrows, Blackbirds	1,550

Figure 47: Partial list of modern birds' relationship and number of species based on DNA analysis (compiled from The Handbook of Birds of the World, volume 1)

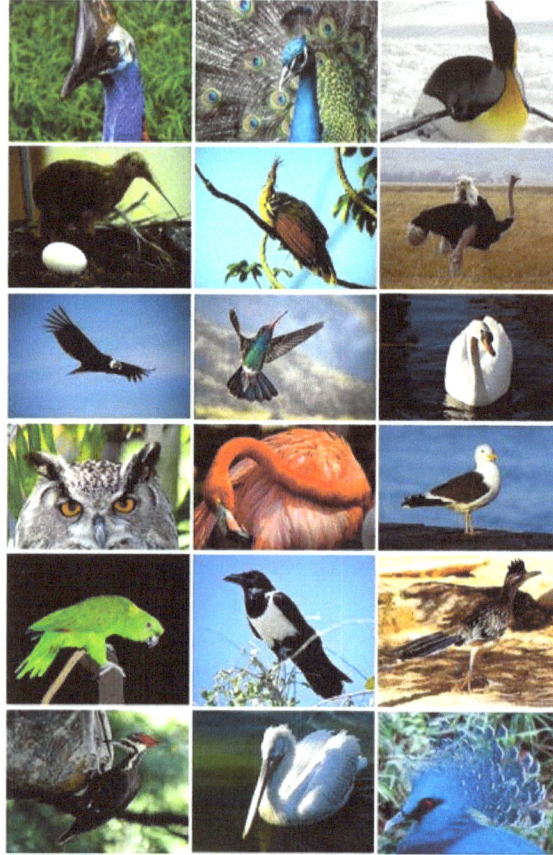

Figure 48: Modern bird diversity (courtesy of wikipedia.org)

Anatomy and Physiology

One of the most significant differences between birds and mammals is flight. Birds possess feathers and in most, hollow bones that enable them to fly. Other significant differences include the absence of a diaphragm, the presence of air sacs and a fused spine.

Feathers

Feathers provide protection for birds and function to enable flight. Feather plumage can also be important for breeding and mate selection. Feather types include:

- Primaries
- Secondaries
- Tertiaries
- Coverts
- Contour
- Tail
- Plumes
- Downy

Primary feathers are found on the ends of the wings, and are generally long narrow and fairly rigid; this functions to provide air resistance and lift during flight. Secondary feathers are found down the length of the wings and provide additional lift for flight. Tertiary feathers are the last feathers on the wing closest to the body and tend to be more ornamental than functional for flight. The shafts of the feathers are covered by small coverts, much like shingles on a roof cover the top of the shingle below it. This overlap provides complete coverage for the bird, and protects the underlying skin. Downy feathers are found under the body and contour feathers and provide insulation and additional protection for the bird. Tail feathers function to steer the bird during flight and are highly variable between species. Plumes, such as the tail plumes of the peafowl, are highly ornamental and are important for breeding and mate selection.

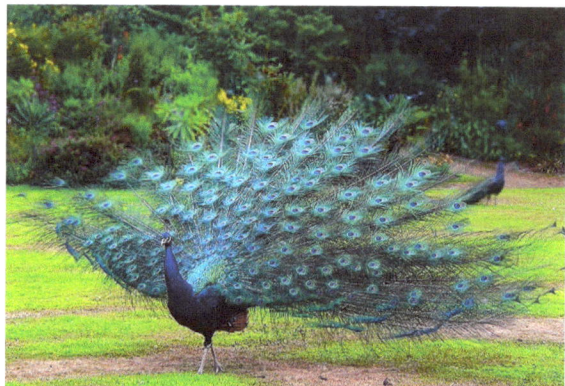

Figure 49: Indian Peafowl male with tail feather breeding plumage. (courtesy of birdsgallery.net)

Feathers are made of keratin, and thus can be considered specialized hair or scales in birds. The feather is made up of the shaft, called the rachis, and the barbs, which make up the surface of the feather. The barbs are made up of

44

interlocking barbules which hold the feather into its shape. Feathers must be groomed and straightened frequently to ensure proper position and function.

Owls have serrations on the leading edges of their feathers; this enables them to fly silently.

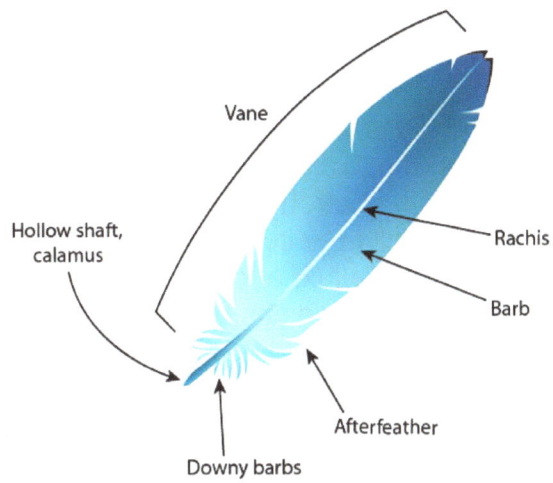

Figure 50: Anatomy of a bird feather (courtesy of askabiologist.asu.edu)

Feathers need to provide weatherproofing and waterproofing for the bird, and therefore must be treated with a special secretion from the uropygial gland, also known as the preen gland. This gland produces oil which birds use to coat their feathers. The uropygial gland is located at the base of the tail in most birds; some species lack an uropygial gland; these include certain ratites, owls, pigeons and parrots. The uropygial gland is well developed in aquatic species such as ducks and pelicans.

Featherless tracts, also called apterial regions, are areas on the bird where no feathering occurs. These areas include the brooding patch under the keel, areas of the flanks, as well as regions on either side of the neck. These areas allow for visualization of the skin, incubation of eggs, or in the case of the apterial region of the neck, allows for visualization of the jugular veins. Columbiformes, like doves and pigeons, is one group of birds that lack some apterial regions including those around the neck.

Moult is the process by which feathers are replaced on birds. Moult can be variable in most species, but generally coincides with breeding seasonality. Many species of birds will moult prior to breeding and once again after breeding season. Some birds will acquire vibrant and highly ornamental feathers during breeding season; this is often the case for male birds, as their ability to breed with a female is often determined by their attractiveness. Moult is not generally a punctuated process; feathers will be replaced as others are being lost. These new feathers are called pin feathers or blood feathers and are highly vascular and fragile during this stage of development. Care should be taken not to damage or cut a blood feather.

The alula is a small feather originating at the carpus of the bird's wing above the first primary feather. It originates from the germinal tissue of digit one. The alula functions to direct airflow over the wing thus increasing lift. The alula is the site for a permanent wing-clip procedure called pinioning in which the germinal bone of the primary feathers is cut. Pinioning is a common procedure for captive bird species in a free-flight setting such as a zoo or open aviary. The patagium is the elastic tissue that connects the carpus of the wing to the shoulder of the bird. The patagium is the site of transponder and identification tags for some species of birds such as California Condors. This area is relatively avascular so it can be easily pierced with rivet-like fasteners; these fasteners can hold ID tags with numbers so individual birds can be identified from relatively long distances. Patagial tags and transponders have enabled researchers to identify and map bird migration and movements as well as nesting and hunting ranges. This information has aided in conservation efforts for some of the most endangered bird species in the world.

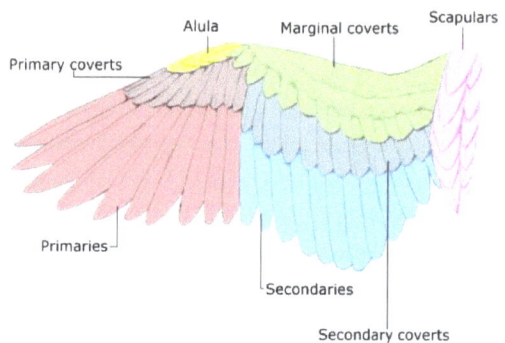

Figure 51: Feather anatomy of the bird wing

Bones

The function of bones in birds is similar to that of mammals; to provide a structure to hold organs, muscles and provide hinges for movement. The ability for birds to fly has resulted in the development of pneumatised or hollow bones. A latticework of interior bone webbing provides strength to the bones. Hollow bones provide a significant reduction of weight to the bird, as well as an increase of oxygen stores. Pneumatised bones are connected to the respiratory system making birds efficient users of oxygen. Some terrestrial birds lack pneumatised bones, and others have varying proportions of hollow bones.

Many of the bones of birds are analogous to those found in mammals; some, however, have been modified to allow for flight.

The orientation of extremities is variable in birds with most having a three toe forward and one toe back configuration. Not all birds have four digits; ostriches and emus have two and three digits, respectively. Digit orientation is based on several evolutionary factors such as food acquisition, grasping and locomotion. The order anseriformes includes ducks and geese that use their webbed digits for movement in water; whereas, the falciformes or birds of prey, use their strong feet and talons to grasp and kill prey items. The rear digit is called the hallux, and serves to oppose the other digits while grasping prey or perching. Digits are counted the same way in other animals with digit one being the thumb or medial digit; the hallux in most species is digit number one.

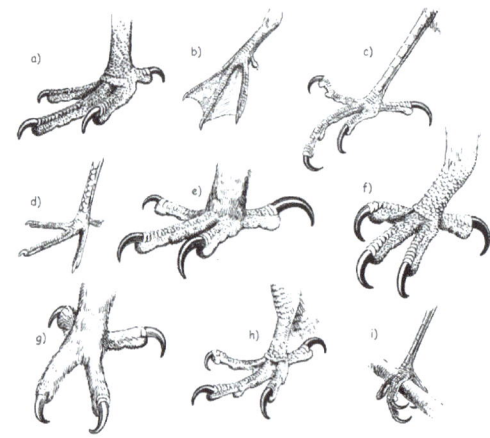

Figure 52: Bird feet types and orientation (courtesy of idahoptv.org)

Foot Type	Number
Anisodactyl	3 forward 1 back
Zygodactyl	2 forward 2 back
Pamprodactyl	4 forward

Table 17: Avian foot orientation terms

46

Bone type	Description
Beak	Made of keritin, the beak conformation enables the bird to eat an appropriate diet; referred to as the upper and lower mandibles.
Keel	Bony structure analogous to the sternum in mammals; it provides attachment for large pectoral muscles.
Furculum	Also known as the wishbone; functions to create spring effect when wings begin upswing during flight.
Pelvis	Large structure analogous to mammals, but fused to much of the spine; little flexibility of the back in birds, but ensures good position during flight.
Spine	Analogous to mammalian spine, but fused to pelvis. Cervical spine long and flexible; as many as twenty-five cervical vertebrae.
Pygostyle	Analogous to coccyx in mammals; contains germinal bed for tail feathers.
Carpus	Analogous to mammals, however, reduced to three digits.
Femur	Analogous to mammals; often covered by feathers and not seen. This gives the appearance that birds' legs bend backwards.
Tibiotarsus	Analogous to the tibia/fibula in mammals.
Tarsometatarsus	Analogous to the metatarsal bones in mammals, however, fused into a single bone.
Phalanges	Analogous to mammals, however, their position can be variable.

Table 18: Bones found in birds

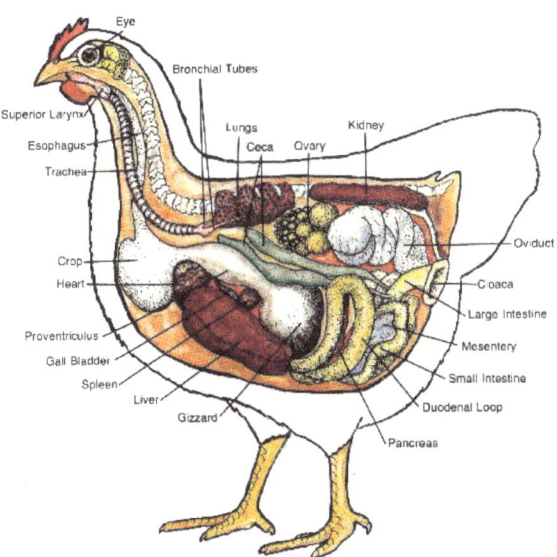

Figure 53: Internal anatomy of a chicken

Respiratory System

The respiratory system in birds is complex and efficient. Due to the metabolic requirements, both the circulatory and respiratory systems must accommodate the physiological demands of flight. Significant differences from the mammalian respiratory system include the presence of closed tracheal rings, a pair of fixed lungs, nine respiratory air sacs and the lack of a diaphragm. Additionally, birds lack an epiglottis like that found in mammals; however, they do have the ability to use muscular contractions of the glottis to close the trachea.

Respiration, as in most mammals, begins at the nasal passages. Birds' nasal passages or nares are generally located at the proximal end of the upper mandible. The nares are found in the fleshy area of some species; this region is called the cere. Some birds possess a small knob-like projection called an operculum within the opening of the nares. The nasal canals terminate inside the oropharanyx at a hole called the choana. The choana is located on the roof of the bird's mouth, and may have a slit-like appearance. When a bird's beak is closed, the choana creates a seal with the glottal opening, hence, connecting the nares to the trachea. Because of this orientation, a bird with open mouth breathing is considered to have an abnormal condition. The glottis can close, but unlike mammals, an epiglottis is not present; mechanical manipulation with a laryngoscope is not necessary in a bird's endotracheal intubation. Birds, however, have closed tracheal rings. This requires special care when intubating birds; cuffed endotracheal tubes are not generally recommended.

Air from the nares passes through the choana and glottis, down the trachea, through the syrinx or voice box and into the lungs. The syrinx is analogous to the mammalian vocal cords and is the source of bird vocalizations. Avian lungs are the site of oxygen exchange, but unlike mammalian lungs, birds have parabronchi instead of alveoli. The presence of nine air sacs in birds further enhances respiratory efficiency. Birds lack a diaphragm to drive respiration. Respiration results from the skeletal movement of the bird which drives air into the lungs and air sacs. Air sacs act as storage for air, and result in air being passed through the lungs twice for every inspired breath.

The respiration process is complex, efficient and worth closer examination. Birds have a pair of lungs, and the following air sacs in most species:

          One interclavicular sac
          Two cervical sacs
          Two anterior thoracic sacs
          Two posterior thoracic sacs
          Two abdominal sacs

The air sacs are thin-walled and act as air storage bags like a bellows; they do not provide gas exchange. The step-by step process is as follows:
When a bird inhales,

Air passes into the lungs and into the posterior thoracic and abdominal sacs.
Air already in the lungs passes into the interclavicular, cervical and anterior thoracic sacs.
Oxygen exchange in the lungs occurs.
When the bird exhales,
Air passes from the posterior thoracic and abdominal sacs into the lungs.
Oxygen exchange in the lungs occurs.
Air that was in the lungs, interclavicular, cervical and anterior thoracic sacs leaves the bird.

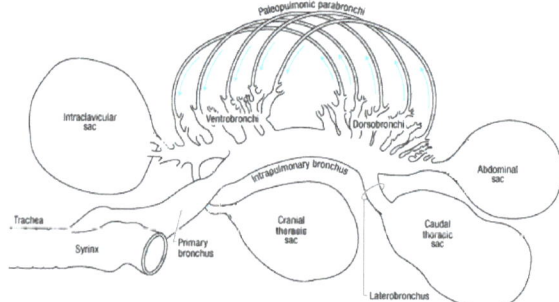

Figure 54: Respiratory model of birds showing lungs and air sacs (courtesy of people.eku.edu)

Respiration in birds should not be labored or difficult; open mouthed breathing should be considered abnormal. Respiration rates can be highly variable in birds and, at times, difficult to assess. In general, as with mammals, small birds will have a more rapid respiration rate than large birds.

For every inspired breath, a bird has two opportunities to have fresh oxygen exchange in the lungs.

Circulatory System

Birds have a four chambered heart like all mammals and crocodilians. Because of their high metabolic need for flight, birds have some specialized circulatory processes. Radiographically, the avian heart is more central in the chest than the slightly left-shifted mammalian heart. Heart rates in birds can be extraordinarily rapid, and in some cases, too difficult to count. In general, just as with mammals, small birds have a higher heart rate than larger birds.

Birds utilize a countercurrent blood flow system to reduce heat loss in their limbs. This is the reason penguins can tolerate standing on icebergs without freezing their feet. Warm core blood is pumped to the extremities via arteries; venous flow returns environmentally cooled blood back towards the heart. Arteries and veins are paired in the limbs allowing for the transfer of arterial heat over to venous return. This heat exchange allows a warming of venous blood before it gets back to the core of the bird.

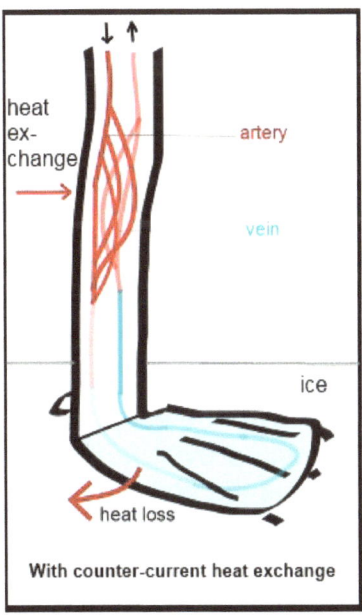

Figure 55: Counter-current heat exchange (courtesy of askanaturalist.com)

The blood morphology of birds is both interesting and unique. The function of blood, however, is the same as in mammals. The differences are as follows:

> Birds possess elliptical nucleated red blood cells.
> Neutrophils in birds are called heterophils.
> Bird platelets, called thrombocytes, are nucleated and function the same as the non-nucleated mammalian platelets.

Red blood cells function to transport oxygen to the tissues of the body. The non-nucleated mammalian red blood cell allows for the bonding of four oxygen molecules per cell. It is theorized that because birds have an efficient respiratory system, the need for extra oxygen molecules on each red blood cell is not necessary.

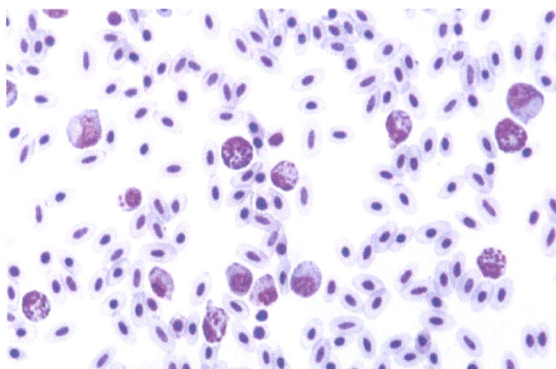

Figure 56: Avian blood smear showing nucleated RBC's and assorted WBC's (courtesy of cvm.ncsu.edu)

Digestive System

The digestive system in birds is similar in function to mammals; the digestive anatomy differs slightly. The digestive system of birds begins at the beak and ends at the cloaca or vent. Whereas, digestion begins in the mouth of mammals by salivation and mastication,

49

birds use their beak mainly for food acquisition.

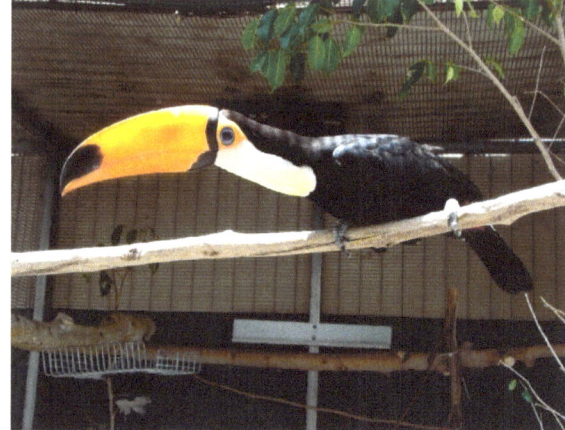

Figure 57: Toucans have large elaborate beaks

Bird beaks are highly variable, but function to pick up, kill or break apart food items. Raptor and parrot beaks are curved and powerful; one for tearing prey items, and one for breaking seeds. Flamingo beaks contain laminae in order to sift food items from the water. Bird beaks, although seemingly strong, are made of lightweight keratin, and can be damaged or broken if traumatized. Bird beaks grow, but are generally worn down by the process of eating and cleaning. Bird tongues are also highly variable and function to acquire food items or manipulate food as it is being swallowed. Some birds use their beaks for food acquisition. Woodpeckers, hummingbirds and lorikeets are some of the birds that make significant use of their tongues for eating. Birds lack teeth, but many species have sharp beak edges and serrations that function as teeth.

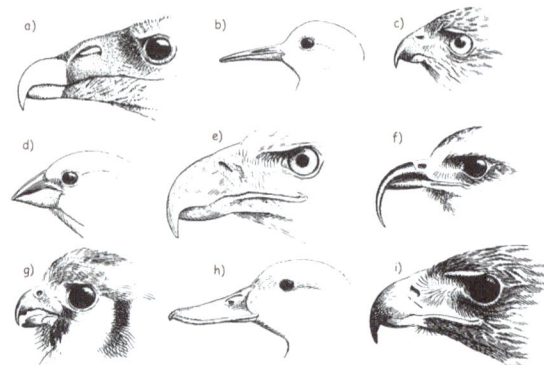

Figure 58: Avian beak types (courtesy of idahoptv.org)

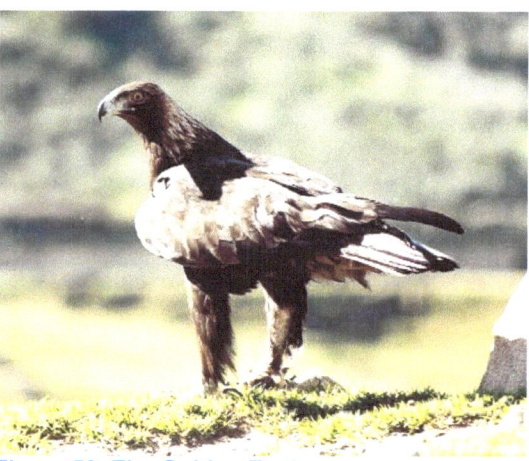

Figure 59: The Golden Eagle

In some birds, swallowed food passes down the esophagus and into a storage container called the crop. The crop enables birds like raptors to gorge on food quickly and digest later. Some birds will hold food in their crop and regurgitate it to waiting chicks, while others will find protection on a roost to continue the digestive process. Crop milk is a special food produced by some birds in their crop and used to feed their chicks.

Food that travels down the esophagus eventually gets to the proventriculus. The proventriculus is the first of a bird's two part stomach. The proventriculus, also called the glandular stomach, is the region where enzymatic food begins to break down. The second part of the stomach, called the ventriculus or gizzard, is where mechanical digestion occurs. Here, food items are ground up with muscular contractions of the ventriculus, similar to what is done in the mammalian mouth with the use of teeth. Some birds ingest rocks and other hard items that they use to help with digestive breakdown of material in the ventriculus. Undigested food items such as fur and bones are sometimes regurgitated in the form of a pellet. This pellet serves to clean the esophagus and crop in many species. Some birds do not produce a pellet.

Digesta from the ventriculus enters the small intestine. Here, with the help of the pancreas, digestive enzymes break-down food, allowing for the absorption of nutrients by the small intestine. Undigested food and waste products enter the very short large intestine and exit through the cloaca or vent.

Bird droppings consist of two constituents; a fecal portion and a urine portion. The feces portion of a bird dropping is generally dark brown or black in color, but can be green, red or a variety of other colors based on the diet of the bird. The urine portion, actually called urates, is white or clear in color and may be present with or without feces. A true 'fecal sample' should include the brown or non-white portion of the dropping. Fecal color and quality is a good indicator of bird health, and should be a part of an avian physical evaluation.

Term	Description
Coelom or coelomic cavity	Body cavity of birds and reptiles due to the lack of a diaphragm
Testes	Internal in birds; become large during breeding season
Phallus	Penis-like structure in some species of male birds including ducks, chickens and ostriches
Oviduct	Female reproductive tract; most birds have a single oviduct
Trachea	Closed-ringed structure connecting the lungs to the oral cavity
Syrinx	Voice box of the bird
Choana	A variable sized slit on the roof of the mouth of birds. The choana connects the trachea to the nares enabling closed mouth respiration
Cloaca	Terminal structure for reproductive and digestive tracts in birds
Proventriculus	Glandular stomach of birds
Ventriculus	Muscular stomach of birds; also known as the gizzard

Table 19: Avian anatomical terms

Reproduction

Propagation is the function of reproduction in all species except some primates including humans. Birds exhibit many interesting reproductive strategies and behaviors. Due to the lack of external genitalia in all birds, sexual differences, known as dimorphism, may not be evident. Other external characteristics may be helpful in determining gender in birds. Some of these characteristics may include the following:

Size dimorphism

In some cases, male birds are larger than females; however, this is the opposite in most raptors. Many birds are similar in size, and in these cases is not a feasible determiner of gender.

Color or plumage dimorphism or polymorphism

Some species of birds have plumage differences that enable gender determination. In general, species that have colorful males also have less colorful and sometimes drab or cryptic colored females. Some birds have colorful plumage only in the breeding season, and at other times are said to be in eclipse plumage, making them virtually indistinguishable from the female of the species.

Vocalizations

Some bird species have unique vocalizations between genders. This may be a valuable determiner in a field setting when the bird may not be seen, but can be heard.

The process of mate selection and reproduction is an important determiner of reproductive success in birds. Simply putting two birds together will not insure propagation. Mate selection is often a female bird decision. Vibrant plumage, vocalizations and ornate displays, are all ways a female bird determines the health of her potential mate. This, in turn, will insure the fitness of her offspring by passing on genetic material from a strong and healthy individual. In some cases, mate selection is made by the type and quality of nest built. The Bowerbird is an example of a bird thats house and yard-keeping are what gets the girl. A lek is another example of a breeding strategy where males protect a defined territory and an interested female enters his territory if it appeals to her.

> Some species have size differences between the sexes.
> Some birds, especially males, develop ornate and colorful plumage during breeding season. Male birds are generally more colorful and ornate than females.

Breeding Strategy	Description
Colonial	Large groups of birds breeding in colonies; monogamous, but polygamy possible. Example: Penguins
Solitary	Individuals that only get together during breeding season. Example: Shoebill
Territorial	Birds that maintain a territory, keeping other individuals out. Example: Golden Eagle
Lek	Male maintains a territory and female chooses mate by entering his territory. Example: Bustards

Figure 60: Breeding strategies of birds

Once mate selection, sometimes called a pair bond, has occurred, many species of birds begin the process of nest building. Some bir'ds nest on cliffs, others in trees and still others simply on the ground. Nests are highly variable in construction and may be a few simple twigs to an elaborate woven house. Many factors are considered when selecting a nest site including proximity to food, direction in relation to the sun and shade, as well as inaccessibility to predators. The process of nest building is generally carried out by both individuals; some birds may even use other birds' nests for their own. Some birds may have several nests in a given territory, using different ones each breeding season, while others may construct a new nest every time. The pair bond is suggestive of monogamy, and some birds are known to mate for life, but polygamy is prevalent in some species, especially those in social and colonial groups.

The male's role in incubation and feeding is variable in birds. Some, like raptors, tend to provide food for both the incubating female, as well as the subsequent chicks. Some male birds do not participate in any of the feeding or incubating; their job is to insure that no other males breed with their female, and therefore, provide protection.

The physical act of breeding in birds, often called copulation, involves the mounting of the female by the male. The female facilitates this by spreading her wings or crouching so the male can position himself on her back. Grabbing the back of the head of the female is common and enables the male to maintain position during copulation. Most male birds lack a true penis, although some, such as anseriformes (ducks and geese) and ostriches, have a phallus. Copulation, therefore, involves the contact of the cloacas of both individuals; this is commonly termed a 'cloacal kiss'. In order for the cloacal kiss to occur, the male must move his tail to the side of the female, and position it nearly underneath her. The act of copulation is a quick process lasting only a few seconds. Anatomically, the single testis of the male produces sperm that is sent out of

the cloaca during copulation. The testes in birds are generally quite small during non-breeding season and grow to over four times their normal size during mating season.

The female reproductive anatomy includes the presence of one or two uterine horns and an oviduct that terminates at the cloaca. The oviduct is the area of egg development. Overall, follicles produced in the ovaries travel down the uterine horns, become fertilized, and travel down the oviduct, at which time a calcified outer shell is constructed. This travel time from follicle to calcified egg can typically take between one and three days.
Once laid, egg incubation in birds takes twelve to seventy-five days depending on species. In general, smaller birds have a shorter incubation time.
Clutch sizes, however, are variable in many species. For example, ducks lay large clutches of up to ten eggs; they usually begin incubation after the last egg is laid. This insures that all of the chicks will hatch at roughly the same time.
Raptors, in comparison, usually lay two to three eggs, initiating incubation after the first egg is laid. This strategy favors the survival of the oldest chick over the younger ones. Double-clutching refers to the production of a second set of offspring in a single breeding season. This can occur as the result of an abundance of food, or if eggs or chicks are lost early in the season. Double-clutching is used by aviculturists to increase production of a given species; eggs of the first clutch are often times artificially incubated.
Depending on the species, offspring will be either altricial or precocial. Altricial species tend to be hairless, or

featherless in birds, and are totally dependent on their parents. Examples include most psittacines (parrots and macaws), columbiformes (pigeons and doves), and most passerines (soft bills). Most raptors (birds of prey) are semi-altricial and are typically covered in white down feathers. Anseriformes (ducks and geese), as well as flamingoes, are considered precocial at hatching and serve a more independent adolescence.

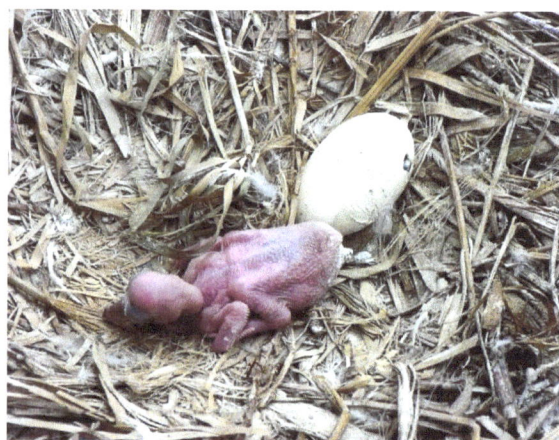

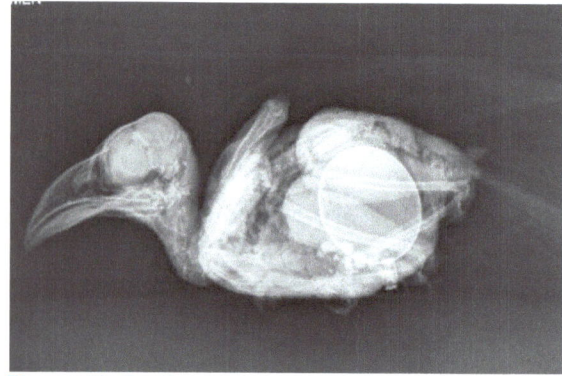

Figure 62: Radiograph of a female bird with egg

Species	Typical number of eggs laid	Incubation period (days)
Golden Eagle	1-3	55
Mallard	8-10	24-28
Scarlet Macaw	2-4	24-25
Cockatiel	3-8	18-21
Sparrow	2	14
Hummingbird	2	12

Figure 63: Egg numbers and incubation periods for assorted avian species

Handling and Restraint

Bird handling and restraint are common and a necessity for some routine medical procedures. Several considerations should be made prior to handling a bird. These include:

- Evaluation of the bird's weapons including beak, talons and spurs.
- The use of restraint devices to limit damage to feathers including the tail.
- The use of minimal but necessary restraint to insure proper respiration of the bird.

Most birds, especially those seen in veterinary practices, have exceptionally strong and sharp beaks as well as strong talons. Birds can be amazingly fast, and once they have you, they may not let go. Caution should be used when working with large macaws, as their beaks have incredible crushing power and may result in finger amputation if bitten.

Nets, gloves and towels are effective ways to approach and capture a bird; these methods may, however, cause unwanted damage to feathers including blood feathers.

Anatomically, birds need to move their skeleton in order to breathe because they are lacking a diaphragm. Careful attention to the bird's respiration during restraint will reduce the likelihood of suffocation.

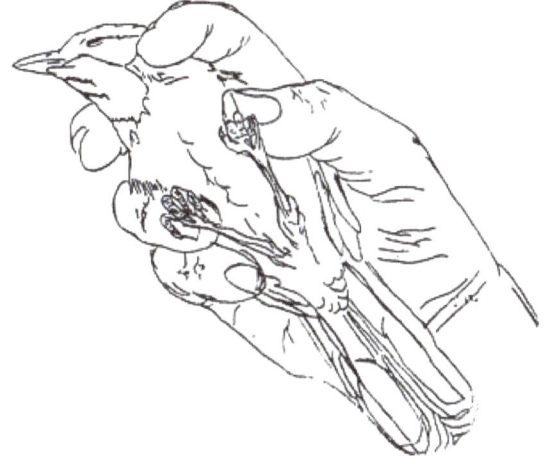

Husbandry

Caring for a bird can be a rewarding and relatively easy endeavor. Most bird species kept as pets include parrots, macaws, budgies, sparrows, mynahs, ducks and chickens. Some falconry hobbyist may have an assortment of raptors including hawks, falcons and eagles. No matter what species is kept, basic husbandry includes the following considerations:

- Proper housing
- Appropriate nutritional diet and water source
- Proper licensing and permits

Housing considerations should include the type and size of structure being used. Birds should have an appropriate sized enclosure or cage to insure the ability to move freely inside without damaging their wings and tail. Some aviculturists may have the ability to provide a large flight cage so birds may exercise and fly-freely without limitations. Branching material in the cage should be of appropriate diameter so the bird can grasp it without sustaining injury to its feet. This can

occur when the branching is too small causing the nails of the feet to wrap around and traumatize the fleshy part of the opposing foot. Toxic plants and branches should never be used in a cage or aviary, and other plants should be evaluated for potential entanglement, traumatic or digestive hazards.

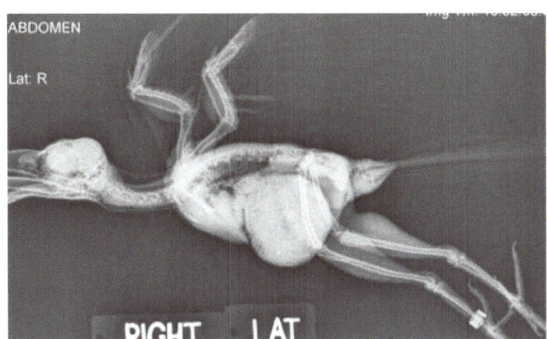

Figure 65: Lateral radiograph showing plant material in the ventriculus of a bird

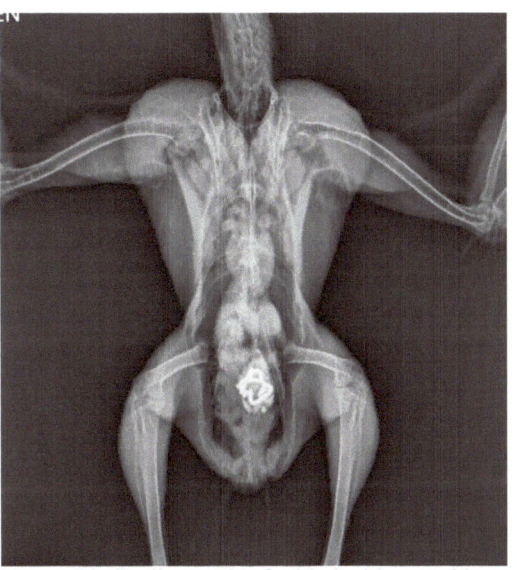

Figure 66: Radiograph of a bird with metal ingesta

Psittacines are notorious for chewing on their cage wiring. Chewing on these wires can lead to ingestion of metal fragments. Zinc is a common alloy found in some cage and wire material; ingestion of this metal can be fatal to birds. Lead, another metal of concern, is generally not seen in cage material, but has plagued California Condors because of their scavenging on animals killed with lead ammunition.

The possession of certain species of birds, especially raptors and other federally protected species, may require permits or special licensing. Falconers are regulated by the Department of Fish and Game, and specific guidelines control the possession of their birds. State or city ordinances may have limitations or permit mandates for the housing of birds in residential areas.

Behavior

Birds, like most animals, will tend to try and escape away from an animal handler; birds will rarely fly towards potential capture. Birds may fan out their wings or put up their hackles (feathers on the back of their neck) when being approached or aggressed. Vocalizations are not uncommon and biting or clawing may occur once the bird is caught. Some birds, on the other hand, may be quite tractable and friendly. Once caught and restrained, most birds tend not to resist.

The art of falconry, also known as the sport of kings, takes advantage of a bird of prey's natural ability to hunt. Falconer's train their birds to hunt for their natural food source, but to always return after leaving the falconer's glove. Cormorants in the orient are used to catch small fish, a normal prey item for the bird. A metal ring is placed on the neck of the cormorant, preventing it from swallowing the fish it catches; the fisherman reels in the cormorant, and removes the fish from the cormorant's mouth.

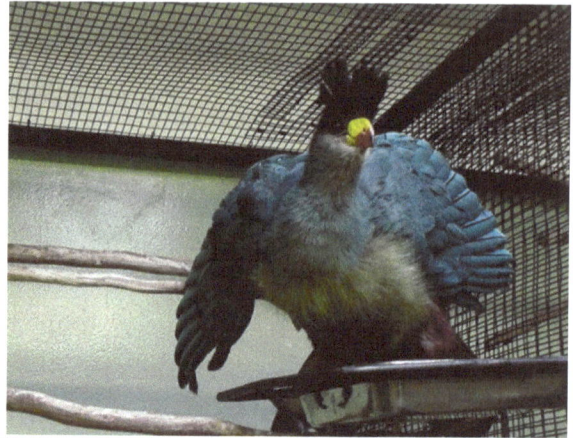

Figure 67: This Great Blue Turaco fans out its wings to look larger and more intimidating as a form of defense

Imprinting

Often seen with ducks and geese, imprinting is a bird's association with a human as its parent. This behavior, usually associated with the artificial incubation and hand-raising of birds, can be both harmless or detrimental. Having a newly hatched clutch of ducklings following you around the yard as if you were their parent has little negative repercussions. An imprinted full grown ostrich or eagle may be more dangerous. Imprinted birds generally perceive themselves as humans, and likewise, are not afraid of people. Additionally, because of this, most imprinted birds are poor candidates for breeding and release into the wild. Conservationists struggle with the need for hand-raising of endangered bird species and the potential for inadvertent imprinting. Many facilities that hand-raise birds use 'feeding dummies' that look like the parent bird to reduce the possibility of imprinting.

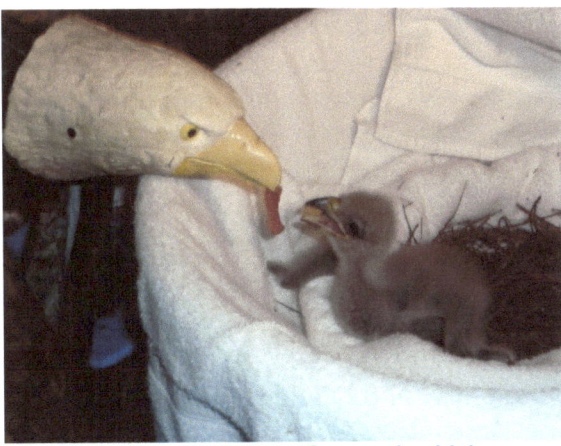

Feeding

Just as with domestic animals, manufacturers of animal diets provide a variety of products for birds. Diets should be specific for the species of bird being kept, and close attention should be taken on food choices by the bird. Some birds prefer selective components of a manufactured balanced diet, and therefore, do not get adequate nutrition. For example, psittacines (parrots, etc) will ravenously eat sunflower seeds, leaving other parts of their balanced diet untouched. These fatty items, by themselves, do not meet the nutritional needs of the bird and can lead to poor conditioning. Natural diets may include fruit, insects or other unique food items a species might eat in the wild. Some hornbills regularly feed on anoles as part of their diet; this food item; however, may not be readily available to the aviculturist. Raptors eat almost exclusively meat, but in a captive setting, may not be provided with enough bones and roughage to provide ideal nutrition. Bones can provide additional calcium to the bird, and roughage can help maintain a healthy crop.

All birds should have access to water. This being said, some birds obtain nearly all of their necessary water from the food they eat. Birds drink by placing their beaks in the water, then raise their heads up and back so the water can run down the throat; columbiformes, which include pigeons and doves, are the only species of birds able to drink by sucking water into the mouth. Water also can serve as a means of bathing for birds, and help maintain healthy and clean skin and feathers.

Common Procedures

The most common medical procedures done on birds include beak and nail trims as well as wing clipping. These procedures can usually be done under manual restraint with little discomfort to the bird.

Nail Trim

Companion animals and birds may require periodic nail trimming. If normal wearing of nails does not occur, nails become long and sharp; long nails are susceptible to traumatic breaking called an avulsion. This condition is a result of the whole nail breaking away from the nail bed and the underlying bone. Significant pain and hemorrhage can occur as a result of an avulsion.

All nails have a blood supply or 'quick' which should be avoided when performing a nail trim. Hemostatic powder, also called quick-stop, can be applied to bleeding nails if needed. Because of the pain involved, cutting a nail to the quick in order to obtain a blood sample should not be undertaken.

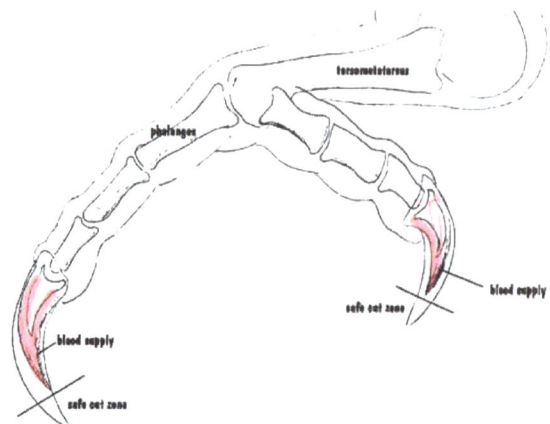

Figure 69: Location of blood supply or 'quick' and safe clipping location for nail trims in birds (courtesy of africangrey.ca)

Depending on the size of the bird, nail trimming can be performed with small human nail clippers, Rescoe animal clippers or motorized Dremel-type cutting tools. Cautery can be used also; it acts to both cut and cauterize the quick in a single cut.

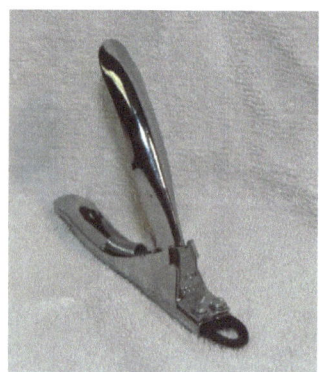 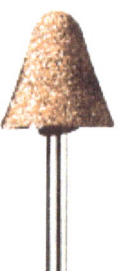

Figure 70: Rescoe nail trimmers (left) can be used to trim bird beaks and nails, and a sanding bit is useful when using a Dremel hand tool.

Beak Coping

Bird beaks are made of the same material as their nails; keratin. A multitude of circumstances may result in the need to trim or 'cope' a birds' beak. Improper wearing down of the beak is the most common reason for a beak cope. During normal feeding, a birds' beak wears down; however, in captive settings, food items may not provide the same kind of wear as in the wild. Additionally, malocclusion of the upper and lower mandibles can lead to improper and unbalanced wearing of the beaks' occlusial surfaces. Poorly balanced diets or metabolic abnormalities may result in rapid beak growth or abnormal beak growth in birds. In these cases, evaluation of the bird's diet and biochemistry profile may be warranted. Always be familiar with the normal appearance of a bird's beak prior to coping.

Wing Clipping

Wing clipping is a technique designed to temporarily render a bird flightless. This technique, however, is not as effective in some species, and must be repeated once new feathers have replaced those that were clipped. The concept is to cut and remove the primary, or flight feathers, so the bird can no longer get lift and fly. The cut is made just above the coverts. Many theories about the best way to clip wings have been described; here is an overview.

Clip the ten primaries on both wings. This is considered the most acceptable method of wing clipping. This does, however, leave both wings symmetrical which can allow some birds to still functionally fly.

Clip the ten primaries on only one wing. This creates an asymmetrical wing conformation for birds that can still fly with both wings clipped. Birds with this clip, tend to circle as they attempt to fly. It has been suggested that clipping only one wing can affect breast and wing musculature due to the asymmetry.

58

Clip all but last two primaries on one or both wings.

Sometimes referred to as a cosmetic clip, some have suggested that leaving two primaries at the end of the wing affords them little protection from damage.

Clip the secondaries in addition to primaries.

This is designed to eliminate additional lift provided by the secondaries. This can be useful in large and wide-winged birds.

No matter what technique is utilized, be aware of any blood feathers and avoid cutting them. Additionally, because blood feathers are at a fragile stage of development, it is best to leave a feather on either side of it for protection. It may be worth having the client return after the blood feather has fully developed. The best wing clip is the technique that works on the individual you are clipping. Optimizing the wing clip of a bird may require several attempts; ask the client what has worked, and what has not worked in the past.

A surgical pinioning can be performed to render a bird permanently flightless, or less flighted. This is a common technique used by zoos and outdoor open aviaries to maintain collection animals without having to handle them for periodic clipping. Some precocial species such as ducks can be pinioned at just a few days of age with minimal discomfort or bleeding. Older birds must undergo anesthesia as this area is more vascular in a mature bird. Scissors can be used on chicks to cut and remove the last two phalanx on the wing. This is located at the bird's carpus; the alula is often used to identify the area to cut. Primary feathers develop from these

bones, and their removal eliminates any feather growth.

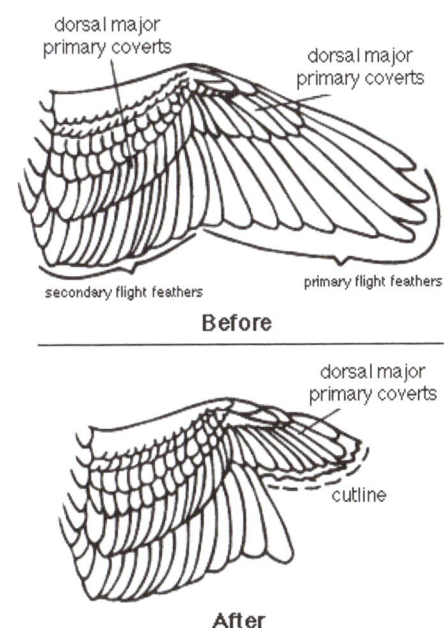

Before

After

Figure 71: Illustration of wing clipping (courtesy of guineafowl.com)

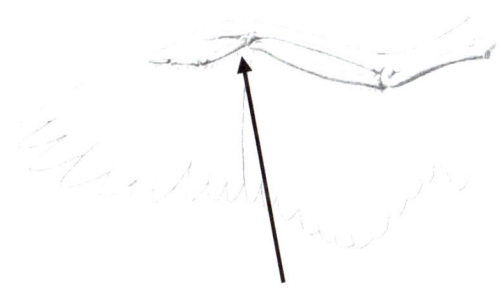

Figure 72: Arrow showing the location of pinion site; the bone is cut and removed at this location.

Wing clipping is a temporary procedure that needs to be repeated after every moult.

Medical Procedures

Most medical procedures on birds can be performed with manual restraint. More invasive or surgical procedures require anesthesia. Most birds tolerate gas anesthetics well; induction and recovery is usually rapid. Ostriches have been immobilized with injectable drugs including ketamine and medetomidine to facilitate handling for medical procedures.

Types of medical procedures may include:

- Physical examination and health certification
- Leg banding and wing tagging
- Beak and wing trimming
- Ectoparasite treatment
- Traumatic injury care
- Sample collection
- Reproductive procedures
- Radiographic imaging

The physical exam of birds should proceed much like that of mammals; a systematic approach from front to back. Many things can be learned about an animal prior to manipulation. Look for fluffed feathers, slouching or other behaviors that are abnormal. If the species vocalizes, the sounds should be clear and free of congestion. Fecal quality can be determined from looking at the bottom of the cage where the bird perched. Once the bird is restrained, the systematic approach may look like this:

- Check eyes for clarity, redness and discharge.
- Check the nares on the beak and the choana in the mouth for patency.
- Check mouth for plaques or discharge.
- Check ears for debris.
- Listen to the heart and lungs for rate, murmurs or congestion.
- Check keel and pectorals for muscle mass.
- Check the wings for symmetry, joint flexibility and feather quality; also check for ectoparasites.
- Check feet for wounds or fractures; determine if nails need to be trimmed.
- Check cloaca for swelling, redness or 'pasty vent'.
- Check tail and uropygial gland (if present) for abnormalities.

Species	Average Weight	Heart Rate	Respiration Rate
Hummingbird	8g	600	120
Sparrow	25g	280	60
Mallard	800g	150	48
Bald Eagle	4,000g	80	24
Ostrich	150,000g	50	16

Figure 73: Physiological values of a variety of birds

Reproductive procedures, such as gender determination, may be necessary for breeding situations when the species are not dimorphic. The laparoscope can be used to look inside the bird and identify the type of reproductive anatomy present. This procedure requires general anesthesia, but requires only one small incision to perform the procedure. Because of this, the procedure is very short, as the bird may require only one suture to close the hole.

DNA sexing can now be performed on a bird using a small blood sample, feather, egg shell fragment or anything that contains sex determining chromosomes. One benefit of this technology is that the bird need not be anesthetized for the procedure.

Egg binding can occur if the egg adheres to the wall of the oviduct during its development. Older birds and birds producing odd sized eggs may be at a higher risk for egg binding. Treatment may include the use of Prepadil, a cervix relaxing gel, or the uterine contraction drug oxytocin. The egg might need to be imploded in order to effectively remove it from the oviduct.

Artificial insemination may be used in some endangered species to insure reproductive success, but overall, AI is not frequently used because of the difficulty in sample collection. Many male birds that are able to contribute semen are often imprinted and uninterested in individuals of their own species. For this reason, many feel natural breeding is far more successful.

Other Medical Procedures

Birds are susceptible to a variety of other medical problems as a result of captivity or the challenges of living in the wild. Car and window strikes can lead to mortality in birds; survivors may have neurologic symptoms or fractures. Birds in captivity may obtain injuries from striking its cage or aviary confines. Some fractious birds may injure their heads in this manner. In all of these cases, triage of wounds and treatment of neurologic symptoms is necessary. Open wounds may require anesthesia and surgical closure to repair. Additionally, the use of crystalloid fluids may be beneficial for birds experiencing hypovolemia due to hemorrhage from wounds. Fluids such as LRS or saline may be prescribed; a five percent of

bodyweight dose is commonly delivered subcutaneously. Heat loss can be a serious problem with sick and injured birds, so warmth in addition to fluid therapy can be helpful in stabilizing avian patients.

Pododermatitis, also known as bumblefoot, is a bacterial condition of birds that results in open abscessed skin lesions on the bottom of the feet. These sores may form as a result of improper perching or substrate that irritates or traumatizes the skin of the foot. Bumblefoot is difficult to treat and resolve because birds are dependent on their feet for standing and in many cases feeding. Treatment of bumblefoot includes the use of antiseptics, systemic and topical antibiotics and anti-inflammatory drugs. Hemorrhoid cream has been used for its ability to reduce swelling.

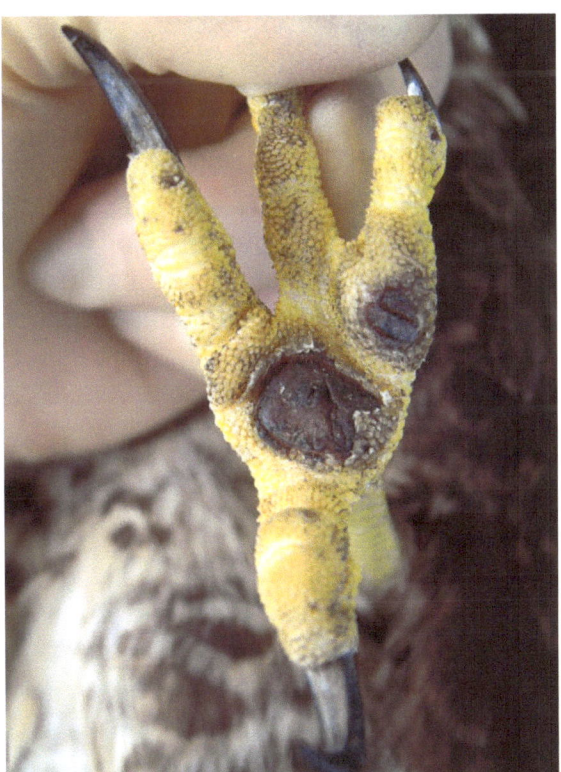

Figure 74: Bumblefoot lesions in a raptor

Compound fractures in birds can be difficult to repair and stabilize; infection and repair failure may occur because it is difficult in many cases, to effectively immobilize the patient. When allowed to heal, bird fractures calcify relatively quickly.

Imping is a procedure used by falconers and bird exhibitors to repair damaged feathers outside of a normal moult. A broken feather may impede flight for a hunting bird; by imping in a feather, this handicap may be minimized. The process involves taking a previously undamaged moulted feather and threading it into the shaft of the broken feather. Cyanoacrylate (crazy glue, Durmabond®) can be used to bond the two feather shafts.

Injections

Routes of injections for birds are similar to those in mammals; most common are subcutaneous, intramuscular and intravenous routes.

Several locations are acceptable for injections in birds. As with all injections, it is important to use proper technique, including aspirating the syringe prior to injecting. Subcutaneous injections can be given in the interscapular space in larger birds; however, the space is much less prominent than in mammals, and may be virtually inaccessible in small birds.

The lateral and medial flanks around the femur are ideal places to give SQ injections because there is much more space in these areas. Additionally, these are featherless areas and simply moving feathers out of the way reveals bare skin underneath. Alcohol or water may be used to dampen feathers in the area to improve visibility. Bird skin can be incredibly thin, so it is important to be careful when giving SQ injections; take care not to overfill fluids in the subcutaneous space as this may tear the skin. The abdominal air sacs reside under the muscle in this area, therefore, take care not to penetrate the needle too deeply when instilling fluids.

Intramuscular injections are ideally given in any of the large muscle bodies of the bird. In nearly all flying species, the breast or pectorals muscles are well developed and are ideal locations for IM injections. Some terrestrial birds may have robust leg muscles; this is an alternative to the pectoral muscles if necessary. Due to the presence of a renal portal system in birds, it is suggested that most drugs should not be injected into the legs if possible. The renal portal system or shunt, is a vascular pathway that can divert blood from the caudal portion of the bird directly through the kidneys before continuing back to the heart. Some drugs may be excreted and damage the kidneys as a result of injecting into the caudal portion of the bird. As with all injections, it is important to aspirate the syringe to insure that the needle is not in a vessel. This becomes especially important when dealing with very small birds.

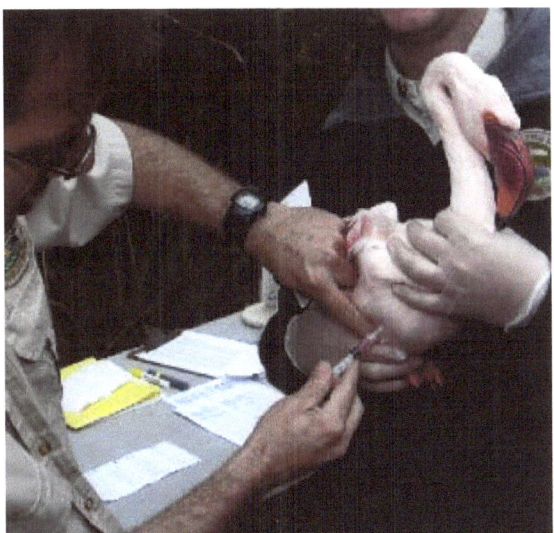

Figure 75: The author gives an intramuscular (IM) injection in the right pectoral muscle of a Lesser Flamingo

Several intravenous injection and blood collection (phlebotomy) sites are present in birds. These vessels include the right jugular vein in the neck, the ulnar or brachial veins of the wings and the tarsometatarsal veins located on the medial legs. All of these vessels are very superficial with little musculature surrounding them. Because of this, bird veins are more likely to hemorrhage (hematoma) after blood sampling. Most birds have a robust jugular vein on the right side of their neck, and a vestigial or absent vein on the left. Additionally, most birds, except the columbiformes and anseriformes, have a featherless area or apterial tract on both sides of the neck making visualization of the right jugular quite easy. Here are two approaches to right jugular venipuncture in birds:

With the bird in an upright position, hold the neck and head with one hand, using the thumb to occlude the vessel. Bridge syringe with hand while taking the sample. This positioning may cause fewer hematoma formations and may be less stressful for the bird. This technique

may require two people with larger birds, but can be done without assistance with small birds if necessary.

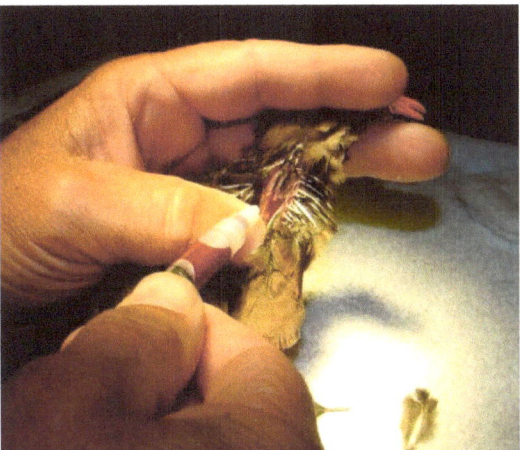

Figure 76: Jugular venipuncture of a bird in upright positioning

With the bird in a left lateral recumbent position, hold the head with one hand, using the finger to occlude the vessel. Bridge the syringe with your hand while taking the sample. This technique always requires two people; one to restrain the bird's body and the other to restrain the bird's head.

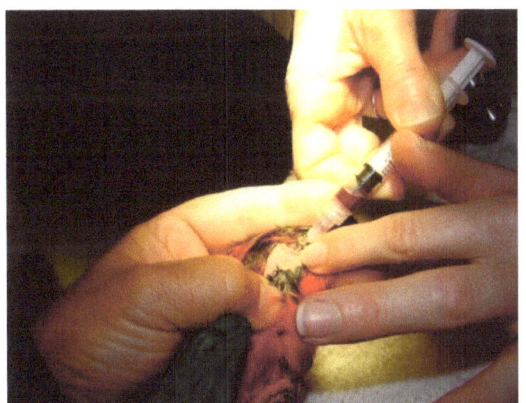

Figure 77: Jugular venipuncture of a bird in lateral recumbency

In most birds, intravenous fluids and blood samples are best facilitated from the right jugular vein.

63

The ulnar or brachial veins are located on the inside of the wings, parallel to the humerus and just distal to the elbow. This vessel rolls over the radius and ulna at its most superficial point. Careful and effective restraint of the bird and its wing is imperative in order to successfully take a sample from this vessel. An assistant typically restrains the bird in dorsal recumbency. The assistant also helps restrain the wing. Post sampling hemorrhage or hematoma formation is very likely at this site, and may require extensive digital pressure or bandaging for hemostasis.

The tarsometatarsal veins are located on the medial aspect of the leg distal to the hock. This vessel can usually be visualized over the hock joint, but may be less apparent further down the leg because of heavier scaling near the foot. To obtain samples from the tarsometatarsal veins, the phlebotomist generally holds the leg while an assistant holds the bird in lateral recumbency. Just as with the ulnar vein, this vessel requires diligent restraint and will likely lead to hematoma formation.

> The Ulnar and Tarsometatarsal veins tend to bleed moderately after sampling blood from them.

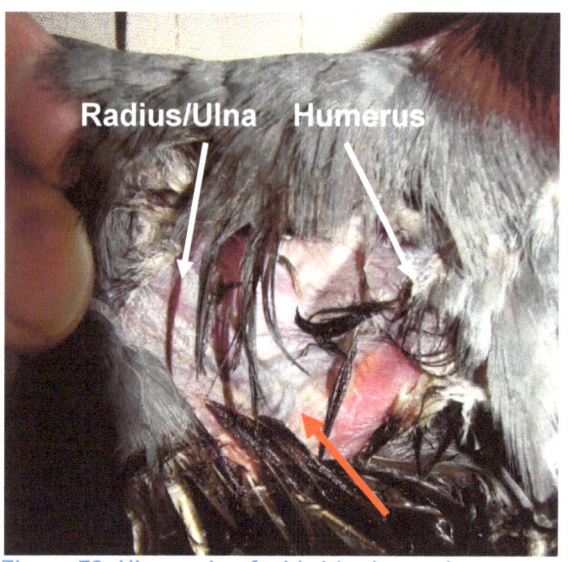

Figure 78: Ulnar vein of a bird (red arrow)

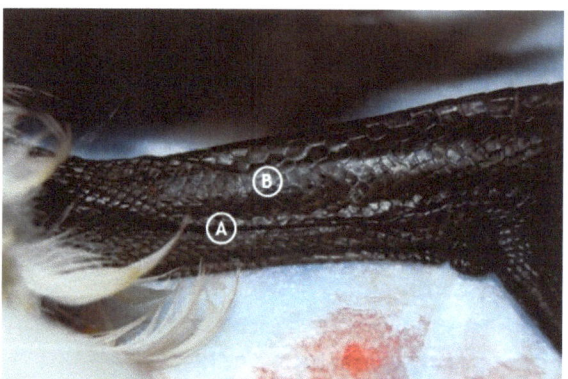

Figure 79: Medial tarsometatarsal vein (A) and TMT bone (B) courtesy of okstate.edu

Subcutaneous (SQ)	Intramuscular (IM)	Intravenous (IV)
Interscapular space (IS)	Pectorals (breasts)	Right jugular
Lateral and medial flanks around the femur	Legs	Ulnar/brachial
		Medial Tarsometatarsal

Table 20: Routes of parenteral administration in birds

The three discussed venous access sites of the bird are acceptable intravenous catheter sites. Of the three, the tarsometatarsal veins offer the most secure area to attach the catheter, and are the least susceptible to catheter occlusion, if properly placed.

Intraosseous catheters can be placed if venous access is unavailable or compromised in the bird. These catheters are placed within the lumen of the bone; here fluid administration can be more easily absorbed into the bloodstream than with the use of subcutaneous fluids. Additionally, fluids can be delivered continuously over longer periods without having to handle the bird. Intraosseous catheters can be placed in any of the long bones of the wings or legs, however, the distal ulna is preferred because of its easy access and limited positioning complications.

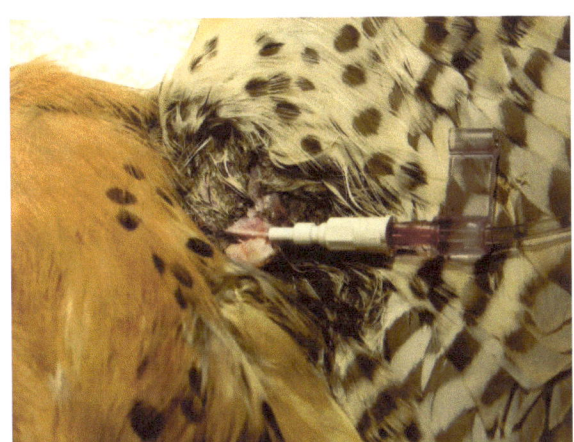

Figure 80: IV catheter placement in the ulnar vein of a Pygmy Falcon

Anesthesia

Anesthesia may be necessary for certain medical procedures in birds. Anesthesia may reduce the risk of injury during procedures such as radiography and wound care. There are, however, restrain devices available that enable

the practitioner to position an awake bird for radiographs; the decision to use anesthesia may simply come down to client cost. Isoflurane is an effective gas anesthetic used for most birds. Because of the efficient respiratory system in birds, gas anesthetic induction, maintenance and recovery are generally rapid. Birds are commonly induced with an anesthetic mask, followed by intubation and maintenance with a gas anesthetic such as isoflurane or sevoflurane. Without stress, most birds can be restrained during the induction process; this can help prevent trauma from thrashing or initial excitatory effects of anesthesia. Risk is inherent to anesthesia, therefore, careful monitoring of patients is essential to minimize complications associated with anesthetic procedures.

Common concerns of bird anesthesia include anesthetic depth, endotracheal tube occlusion and respiratory quality.

> Monitor bird anesthesia closely for changes in respiratory rate and quality....these changes may indicate trouble

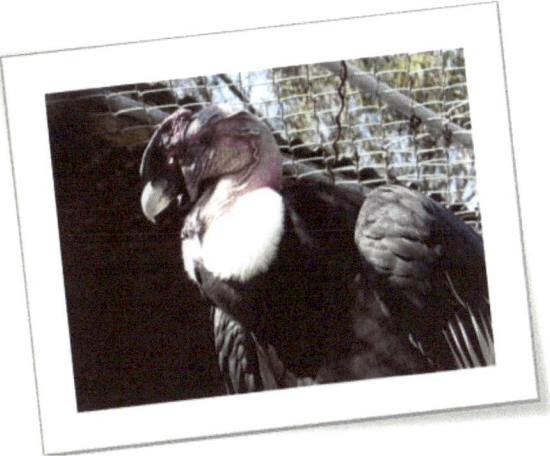

Andean Condor

Anesthetic Concern	Reason	Solution
Anesthetic depth	Anesthetic depth is maintained at about 2.5% isoflurane in most species	Some birds may require more or less anesthesia based on species, age or health
Endotracheal tube occlusion	Endotracheal tube lumen is small for some birds	Periodically provide 'sigh' breaths to insure tube is not occluded
Respiratory quality	Anesthetic depth and time will affect respiratory quality	Careful monitoring of respiration rate and reduction of anesthesia if needed

Table 21: Bird anesthesia concern

Anesthetic dynamics change rapidly in birds. Careful monitoring of birds under anesthesia should be performed by qualified individuals and anesthetists. Veterinary support staff can help by noticing initial changes in anesthetic factors that lead to mortality.

Intubation

Intubation is an effective way to create a patent airway during anesthesia for any species of animal. Birds can also benefit by intubation in longer surgical procedures. In some cases, intubation is a time consuming additional step in a normally short anesthetic procedure. Furthermore, some birds can be difficult to intubate because of their small size or limited visualization of their glottis. Normal lubricants of the tracheal lining also, can cause endotracheal tube occlusion with small birds.

Because birds lack an epiglottis, the use of a laryngoscope is not needed. Intubation in birds simply requires opening of the mouth so the glottis can be visualized. The endotracheal tube for birds is designed to seat against the glottal opening and prevent air 'blow-by'. Because of the closed tracheal rings in birds, cuffed endotracheal tubes common for use in mammals should be used with care by trained individuals. In birds, tracheal damage can occur with misuse of snug or cuffed endotracheal

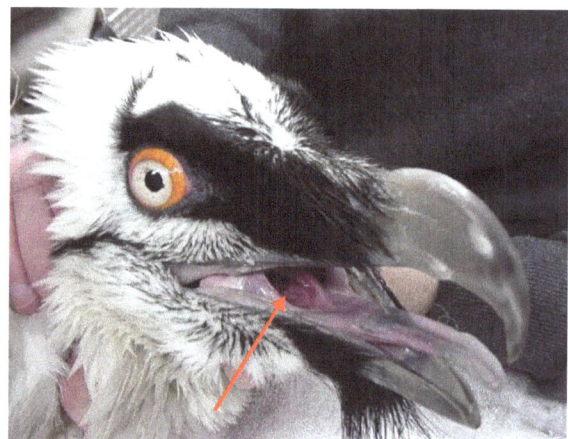

Figure 81: The Bearded Vulture or Lammergier showing a large glottal opening (arrow)

tubes. Occlusion of endotracheal tubes can occur with small species of birds. Endotracheal tube types commonly used include the Cole tube and Cook tube. These tubes are generally wider at the top of the tube, and taper down towards the end. Cole tubes range in size from 8mm to 18mm inside diameter; Cook tubes are 1mm and 1.5mm. Polypropylene IV catheters (without the needle stylet) can be fashioned as endotracheal tubes for very small patients. These tubes can be more rigid than other types and could cause kinking or occlusion of the tube against the tracheal wall.

66

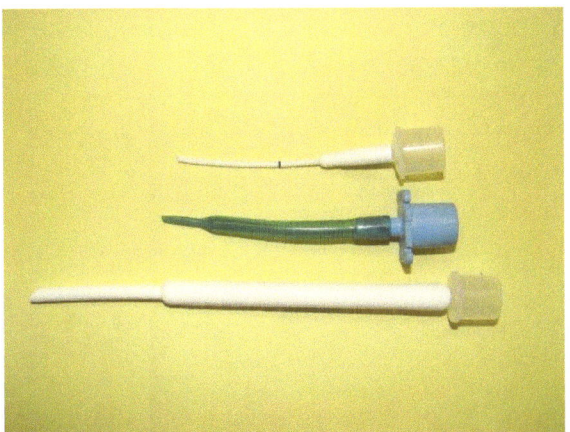

Figure 82: Cook endotracheal tube (top) and 2 Cole endotracheal tubes used for bird and reptile intubation

Endotracheal tubes for birds can be secured with tape either around the lower or upper beak, or around the back of the head. Taping the endotracheal tube around the head tends to be a more secure method and results in fewer unwanted extubations from tape failure around the beak.

Ventilation
Birds are very efficient breathers and tolerate gas anesthetics well. Periodically, assisted ventilation may be necessary to expand the lungs or determine endotracheal patency. This procedure is called a 'sigh' breath, and is useful during long anesthetic procedures in all animals including birds.

Mechanical Ventilation
The advent of pediatric ventilators and small animal ventilators for research medical facilities has benefited birds as well. Mechanical ventilation is a great way to ensure patient respiration and prevent endotracheal tube occlusion. Additionally, the use of a mechanical ventilator reduces the amount of anesthetic gas needed to maintain anesthesia.

	Anesthetic setting for Isoflurane	Anesthetic setting for Sevoflurane
Induction	4-5%	8%
Maintenance*	1.5-2.5%	3-4%
Recovery**	0%	0%
*some species such as columbiformes may require higher maintenance levels of gas anesthetics; some may need more or less based on excitement, health, respiratory quality or degree of pain		
**most species arouse faster if medical oxygen is transitioned to room air shortly after recovery is initiated, as increased CO_2 levels and lower O_2 concentrations help drive respiratory action.		

Table 22: Anesthetic machine settings for birds

Surgery
Birds tend to have fewer elective surgeries; spays and neuters are uncommon in birds. Injuries that may require surgery for a bird include wounds, fractures and egg binding. Traumatic injuries may occur as a result of aggression with other individuals, collisions or hazards inside cages or housing. This may result in lacerations of the skin requiring surgical closure. Fractures can occur most commonly from collisions with objects; fractures have been seen in wild birds as a result of gunshot while flying.
Egg binding can occur as a result of adhesions during the process of egg production. Surgery is necessary once non-surgical methods of egg removal have failed.
In all surgical cases, and just as with mammals, careful attention to vital signs and management of heat loss is important to improve patient survival.

Diseases
Several diseases are of concern in birds. Some involve the respiratory system, while others affect the bones,

feathers and skin. Some diseases are highly contagious to other birds, and some are zoonotic. Treatment for some diseases includes medicines; some can be prevented with vaccination. Birds can be very stoic, and therefore may not appear to be sick. Diagnostic tests and evaluation of early behavior changes can be very helpful in identifying diseases in birds. Sick birds may appear 'fluffed', have poor feather quality, be inappetent and produce discolored or malodored feces. Some diseases, like aspergillosis, are obtained from the environment, while others are highly contagious and are obtained from other individuals. Stresses of captivity and confinement may be attributed to increased disease susceptibility.

Aspergillosis is a fungal disease found in moist soil. Because it is readily prevalent in the environment, aspergillosis is believed to afflict birds in stressful conditions where their immune system may be compromised. Respiratory symptoms such as dyspnea and audible respiratory noise are common in birds with aspergillosis. Symptoms may take time to fully develop, but inappetence, fluffed appearance and exercise intolerance can be indicative of early disease. Acute symptoms may be the result of an aspergilloma occluding the airway. These aspergillis masses are difficult to remove and tend to produce a grave outcome. The placement of an airsac cannula can help bypass the obstructed airway as a lifesaving measure. In general, however, due to a bird's complex respiratory system, aspergillosis is very difficult to treat to resolution.

Diagnosis is made with survey radiographs and diagnostic blood tests looking for aspergillosis antibodies. Treatment of aspergillosis includes the use of systemic antifungal drugs and airway nebulization.

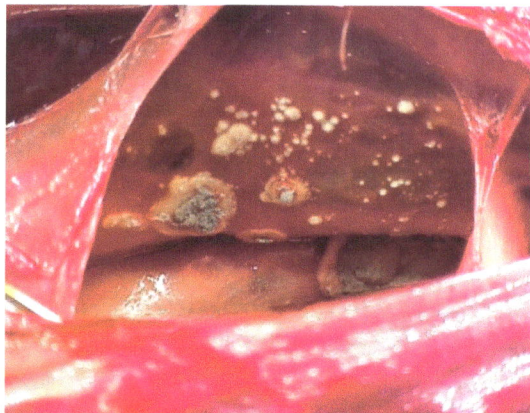
Figure 83: Aspergillosis fungal lesions in the air sac of a bird

Cryptococcus is a fungal disease spread to other animals by infected bird feces. Respiratory symptoms may be present, as well as cutaneous lesions. Cats are more likely than other species to acquire the disease from ingesting contaminated feces. Diagnosis is made from clinical signs and identification of the organism on cytology. Treatment includes the use of antifungal drugs.

Psittacine Beak and Feather Disease (PBFD) is a viral disease affecting mostly young birds in the psittacine family. Findings include feather loss, poor feather development and feather pigment changes. Immunosuppression is also evident. Diagnosis is made from clinical appearance, blood tests and follicular biopsies. The disease is highly contagious and usually requires isolation and euthanasia of affected birds.

Chlamydiosis is a bacterial disease of psittacines and is also known as

68

ornithosis, psittacosis and parrot fever. The disease is spread by inhalation, but transmission to mammals can occur from the ingestion of contaminated birds. Chlamydophila psittaci presents a zoonotic potential and can be a concern when working with birds, especially in large bird farms and slaughterhouses. Symptoms include fever, chills, pneumonia, nasal discharge, inappetence and diarrhea. The disease is treated with antibiotics such as Tetracycline and Doxycycline.

West Nile is a mosquito vectored viral disease affecting birds and mammals. Some bird species such as crows, jays and raptors are highly susceptible and are used as sentinel species. Affected birds may not appear sick while others will succumb rapidly. Symptoms include neurologic and flu-like signs; blood tests can determine the presence of antibodies for the virus. Some birds may not appear sick and are considered carriers. West Nile has a zoonotic potential with similar symptoms in humans. Supportive care for secondary symptoms is the only treatment for affected birds. Prevention includes the elimination of mosquito breeding areas such as ponds with standing water. Vaccines are available for the prevention of West Nile virus in horses; the product has been used off label in birds with some promise. California Condors are vaccinated against West Nile virus due to their high profile endangered status.

Malaria is a disease obtained from one of several protozoan parasites in the plasmodium family. The disease is transmitted by mosquitoes and is treated with anti-malarial drugs. Affected birds become weak, depressed,

anorexic and anemic, while others may be asymptomatic. Parasites can be seen on prepared blood smears or evaluated with serologic testing.

Avian poxvirus is a highly contagious viral disease transmitted by contaminated substrates and mosquitoes. The disease is characterized by visible wart-like lesions and crusty scabs around the beak and legs. Treatment includes isolation of affected birds and antibiotics for secondary bacterial infections. Mortality is high in affected birds. Vaccines are available and used in the poultry industry, but its efficacy in wild birds has not been determined.

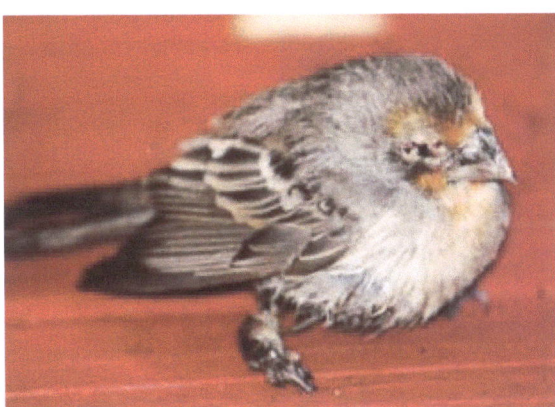

Figure 84: Sparrow with pox lesions around the eyes and feet (courtesy of birds.cornell.edu)

Avian tuberculosis is an infectious disease of birds caused by one of three acid fast mycobacterium bacteria; the other two affect bovid and humans. The disease, spread by inhalation, affects the respiratory system. Tubercles form in the lungs and spread to other organs and cause general malaise, fever, anorexia and dyspnea. Diagnosis in birds can be made with radiographic imagery; lytic bone lesions are characteristic of advanced pathology.

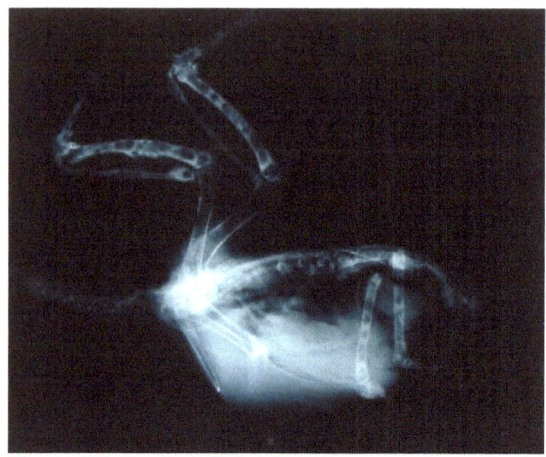

Figure 85: Radiograph showing lytic TB lesions in wing and leg bones of a pigeon

Treatment can include the use of long term antibiotics and supportive care, but in many cases, due to the contagious nature and significance of the disease, euthanasia is often recommended.

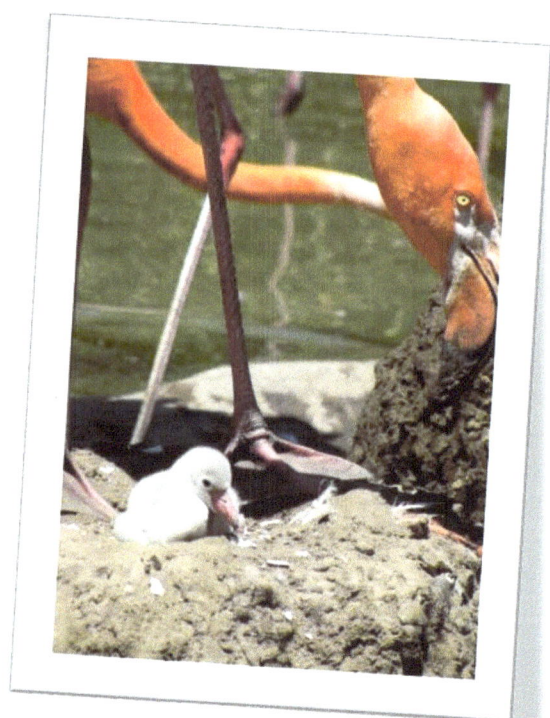

Caribbean Flamingo and chick

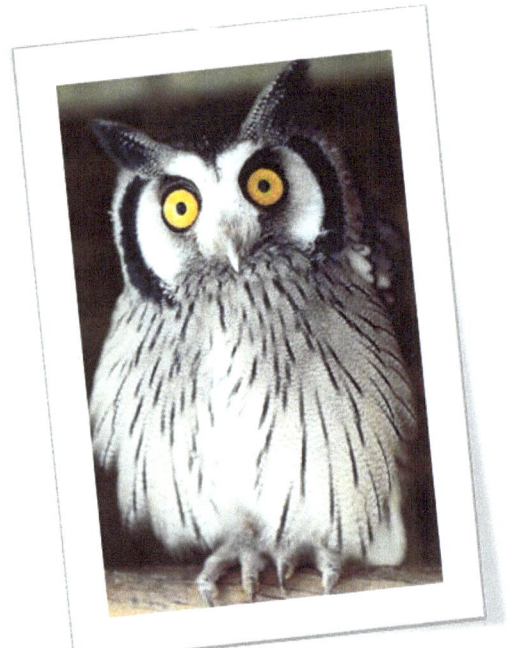

White-faced Scops Owl

Reptile Medicine

Reptiles are a diverse group of terrestrial and aquatic animals. They are grouped into the following taxonomic orders:

- Crocodilia (alligators and crocs)
- Sphenodontia (Tuatara)
- Squamata (snakes and lizards)
- Testudines (turtles and allies)

Reptiles are distinguished by several characteristics including ectothermy.

A reptile's body temperature changes according to the environmental temperature. Ectotherms are also referred to as 'cold blooded' animals. Reptiles are also known for their scaled and armor plated body coverings, which are shed periodically. Yearly shedding enables reptiles to continue growing in length and girth. This is a cycle that continues throughout their lives. This ability is not shared by mammals. Reptiles, however, have the ability to breathe like mammals, using lungs not gills.

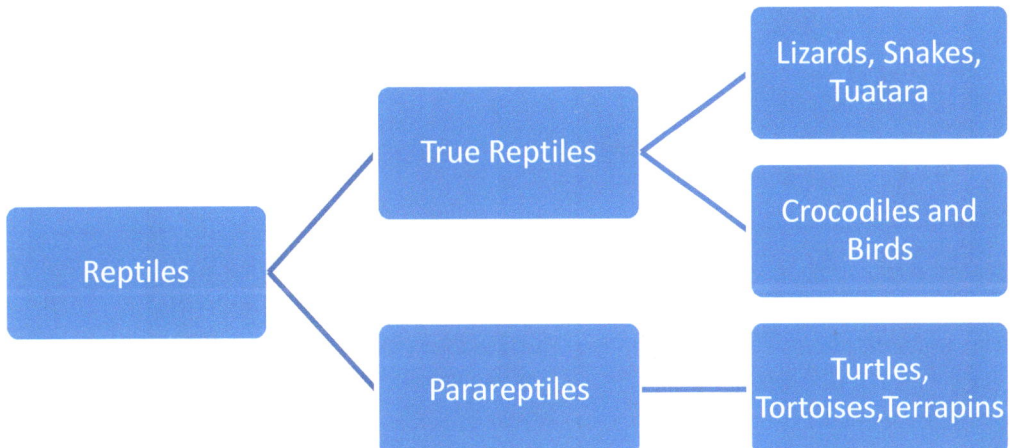

Table 23: Relationship between living reptiles

Order	Types	Species	Habitats
Crocodilia	Crocodiles, Gharials, Caimans and Alligators	23	Freshwater lakes, ponds and swamps of southern United States and China (Alligators), and freshwater lakes, streams and brackish waters of Africa, Australia, Asia and the United States (Crocodiles)
Sphenodontia	Tuatara	2	Exclusive to New Zealand
Squamata	Snakes and Lizards	9,100	Aquatic and terrestrial species on every continent except Antarctica
Testudines	Turtles, Terrapins and Tortoises	300	Aquatic and terrestrial species on every continent except Antarctica

Table 24: Reptile orders, species numbers and habitats

Term	Definition
Brumation	Cooling, usually artificially, to initiate hibernation or wintering
Cloaca	As in birds, the terminal point of excretory and reproductive tracts
Crepuscular	Feeding or active at dusk and dawn
Disecdysis	Difficult or incomplete shedding of scales (see ecdysis)
Ecdysis	Normal shedding of scales
Gravid	Pregnant, or containing eggs
Hemipenes	Male reproductive structures analogous to penis in mammals
Hook	Curved stick used to immobilize or restrain snakes
Jacobson's Organ	Sensory organs of smell found in front of the roof of the mouth in reptiles
Mental groove	Separation in front lower jaw of most snakes that allows for expansion while swallowing large prey items
Oviparous	Egg laying species
Ovoviviparous	Live birth laying, however eggs are carried within the reptile; there is no parental/fetal contact
Parthenogenesis	A form of asexual reproduction found in a few reptile species where embryonic growth and development occurs without fertilization
Retained eye cap	Scale over eye does not shed during normal ecdysis
Spur	Found in Boas and pythons, bony protrusions near the cloaca that are vestigial hind limbs
Viviparous	Live bearing species; mother and fetus blood supply and nutrient exchange are connected

Table 25: Reptile terms

Anatomy and Physiology

Reptiles possess several unique anatomical and physiological characteristics when compared to mammals. When comparing these processes, it is important to consider the habitats, metabolism and thermoregulatory strategies of the species. Reptiles are more closely related to birds when considering their similarities in anatomy and physiology. For example, both birds and reptiles have scales, lack a diaphragm, have a cloacal opening and in most cases lay eggs. Birds have been described as specialized reptiles.

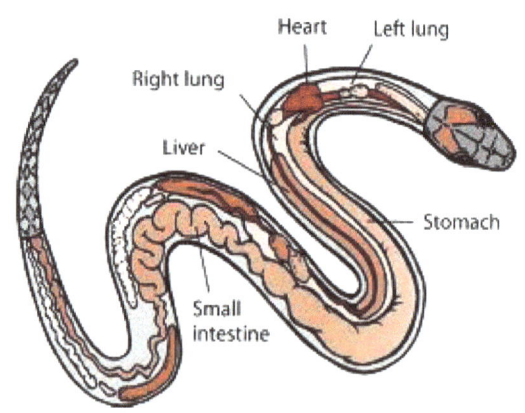

Figure 86: General snake skeletal and internal anatomy

72

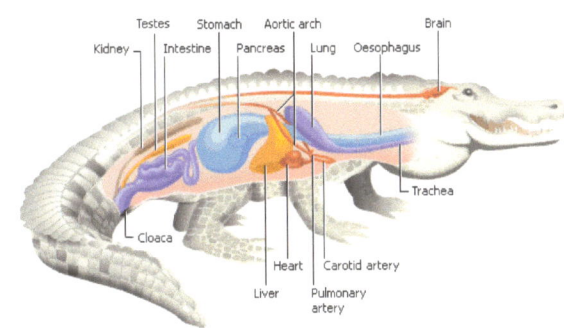

Figure 87: Crocodilian internal anatomy

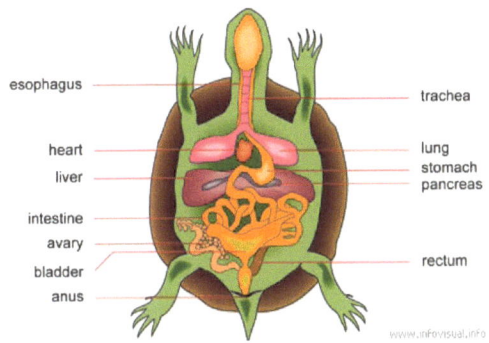

Figure 88: Turtle internal anatomy

Integument or Skin

Reptile skin is covered in thick epidermis; this layer is often covered with bony scales and armor-like plates. Scales and scutes help protect reptiles while affording protection from predators and the environment. The dermal layer of skin in reptiles is thin compared to mammals. Reptile skin is watertight and enables them to easily inhabit aquatic or terrestrial environments. Shedding is the mechanism in which reptiles enable themselves to grow. Snakes and lizards will shed their skin periodically; snakes are known for shedding their skin in a single tube-like piece. Shedding can be a challenging time for both reptiles and handlers; it is sometimes referred to as 'turning blue' and is characterized by a bluish hazing of the skin. During this time, the underlying new skin is fragile and easily damaged with improper handling. Additionally, as the scales on

the eyes (eye caps) are shed, snakes can have decreased visual acuity and may strike handlers inadvertently. Turtles and tortoises shed less regularly than other reptiles, and most will build up layers of scutes on their shell or carapace.

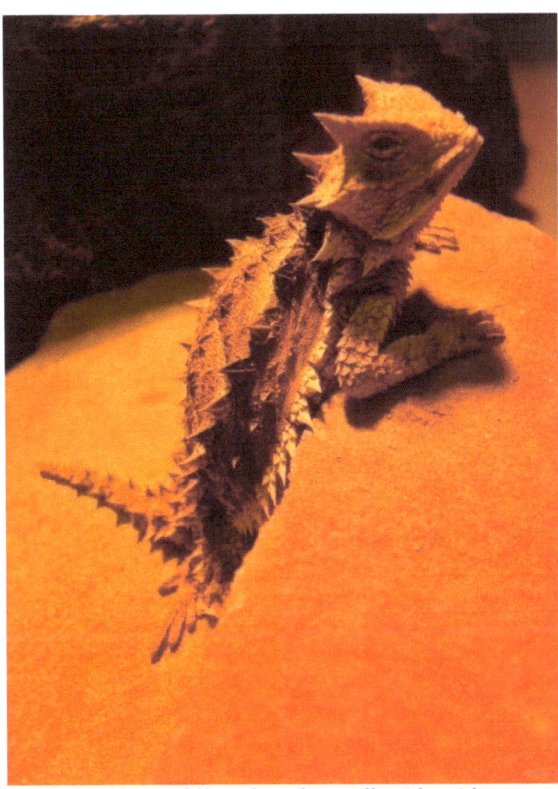

Table 26: Horned lizard under radiant heat lamp

Skeleton

The reptile skeleton is similar to other species of animals, although, due to their ambulation they have limited limb mobility. Snakes lack legs, but instead, have ribs the whole length of their bodies. Additionally, snakes have dislodgeable jaw bones that enable them to engulf large food items. Turtles and tortoises have a fused vertebral column attached to their shell or carapace, and their sternum is wide, forming into the bottom of their shell or plastron. Reptiles can suffer from calcium deficiencies, making them candidates for metabolic bone disease.

73

This can cause folding fractures of the bones; it can be further compounded by egg laying and the abundant calcium requirement needed for shelling eggs.

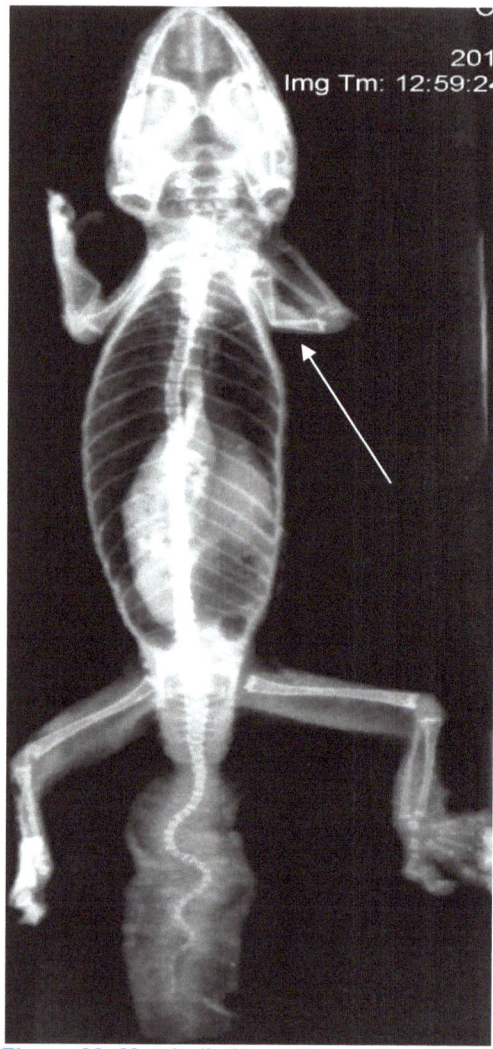

Figure 89: Metabolic bone disease in a lizard, note folding fracture of left humerus (arrow)

Some lizards are able to 'drop' their tail as a means of distracting predators. This process, called autotomy, allows lizards to flee while the predator is fascinated by the lizard's wiggling tail. Autotomous lizards are able to re-grow their tail to nearly its original length; re-growth occurs from the germinal tissue at the fracture line of the tail.

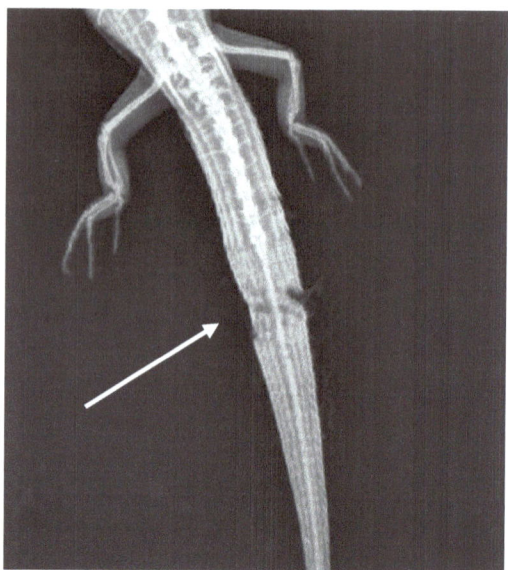

Figure 90: Fracture line of autotomous lizard

Circulatory System

The metabolic needs of most ectotherms are low relative to their endothermic counterparts. Reptile activity and relative environmental temperature dictate the need for tissue perfusion nutrient delivery and oxygen exchange. Because most reptiles are 'lie and wait' predators, their metabolic needs tend to be low. In general, reptile heart rate, respiration rate and temperature are lower than comparably sized endotherms. Even though reptiles have a heart and lungs, these organs have functional differences from endotherms.

The heart consists of two atria and a single ventricle. This three chambered heart functions the same as the mammalian four chambered heart, however there is a significant difference. In the reptilian heart there are two atria, but only one ventricle. Because of this, venous blood returning to the heart is mixed with arterial blood returning from the lungs. And upon ventricular contraction, ventricular 'mixed' blood is ejected to both the lungs and into circulation. The septum found in the mammalian heart separates venous and arterial blood flow, making the system more efficient. Crocodilians have a four chambered heart like their bird cousins; this is due to the common ancestry they share. Functionally, it is believed that crocodiles do not require a four chambered heart, but because they do, the heart beats more efficiently; hence, they grow larger than other reptiles. Additionally, crocodilians are able to stay submerged for longer periods because they can make better use of their circulatory system and blood flow pathways.

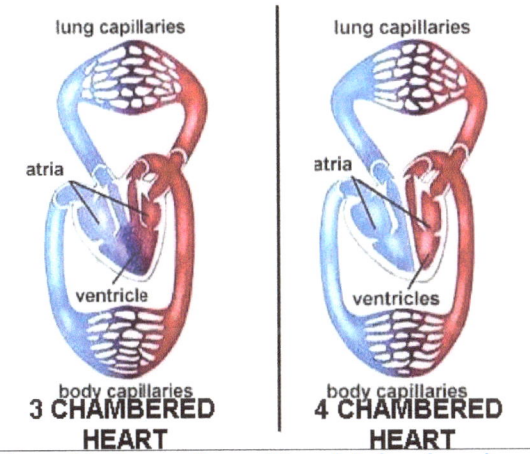

Figure 91: Comparison of 3 and 4 chambered heart anatomy

Digestive System

Depending on the species, reptiles can be considered herbivorous, insectivorous, carnivorous and omnivorous. Unlike birds, all reptiles, except turtles and tortoises, have teeth to aid in acquisition and mastication of food items. Some dentition is small and ridged, and others have fanged teeth for injecting venom into prey items. Digestion is generally a slow process, and some reptiles may eat infrequently. The digestive tract of reptiles terminates at the cloacal opening; feces are often malodorous with white and clear urates.

Reproduction

With the exception of parthenogenesis, reproduction in reptiles is sexual. Anatomically, the act of copulation is similar to that in birds: the cloacal kiss. Unlike in birds, however, male reptiles are equipped with two penile-like structures called hemipenes. One of the two hemipenes is inserted into the female's cloaca during copulation. After copulation, the male's role in parental care is minimal or absent. In many cases, the female's role ends after egg laying. Unlike birds, egg laying reptiles do not incubate eggs; more often, they will guard over them or bury them and leave.

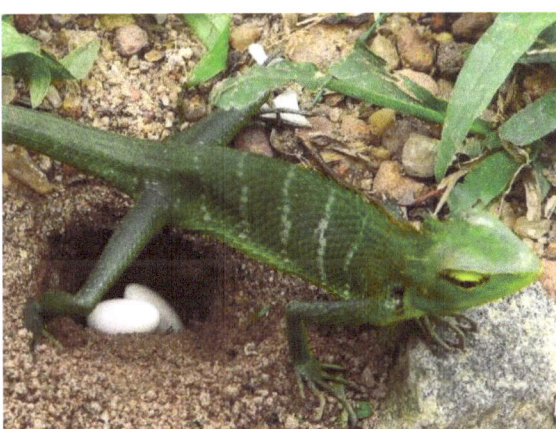

Figure 92: Lizard laying eggs

Handling and Restraint

Reptiles come in many forms with a variety of armor plating and sharp scaling. Additionally, reptiles have sharp crushing teeth, with some reptiles having dangerous and toxic venom. These cold blooded and seemingly slow animals are amazingly agile and potentially harmful if not handled with respect. Here are some considerations prior to handling a reptile:

75

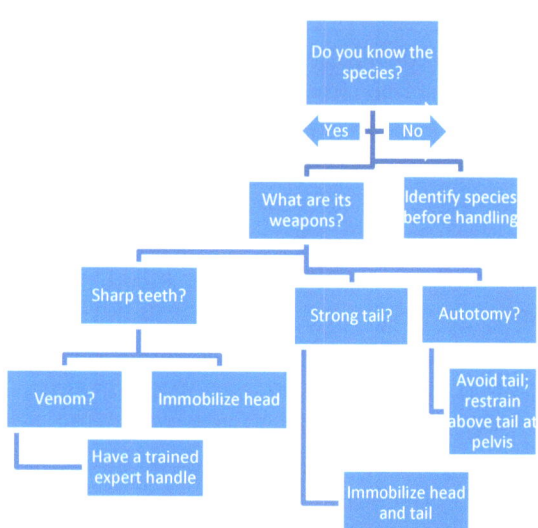

Table 27: Systematic approach to reptile handling

It is very unlikely that a venomous reptile will be brought to a veterinary practice; however, all reptiles should be treated as potentially venomous until their species is identified.

Most reptiles can be restrained with minimal effort; some may require more strength and protective equipment. Types of protective equipment used in reptile restraint include gloves, towels, snake hooks and plastic snake tubes. Turtles and tortoises can be restrained simply by lifting them off the ground; larger specimens can be balanced on a block of wood or a bucket. If at all possible, avoid placing a turtle or tortoise on its back.

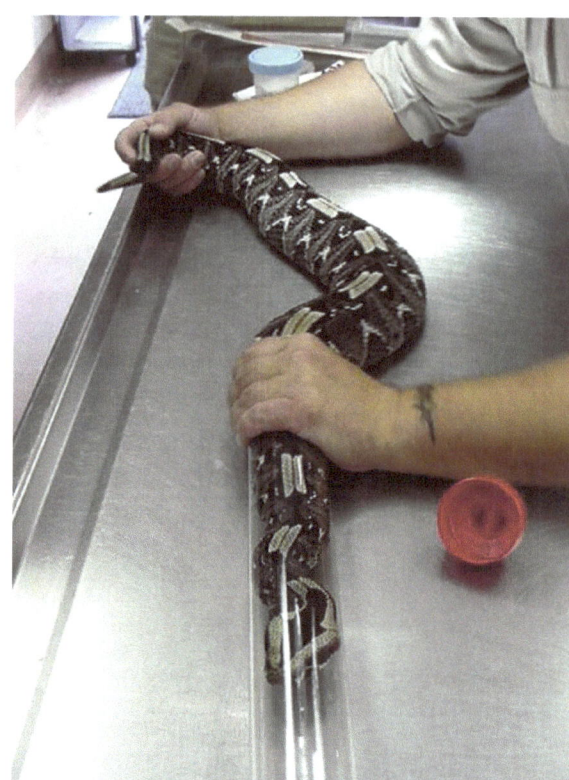

Figure 94: Snake tube for venomous snake restraint

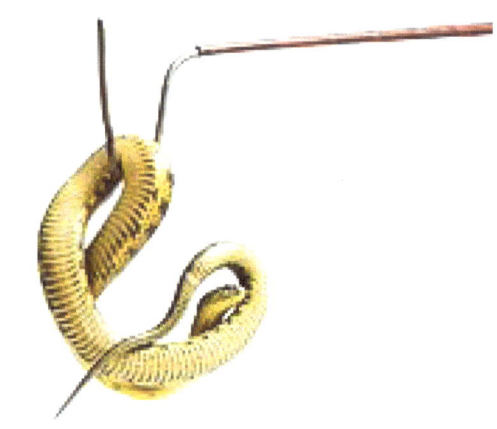

Figure 95: Snake hook

Some lizards relax as a result of light digital pressure over both eyes; this can be used to position and reduce movement of a lizard when it is necessary to take a radiograph.

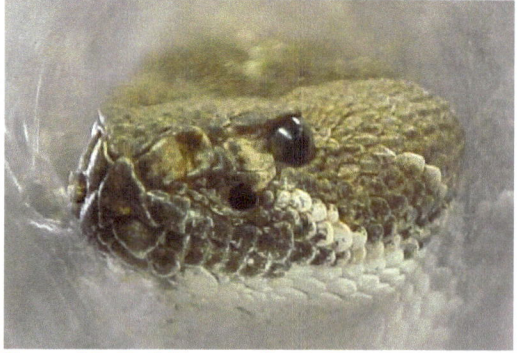

Figure 93: Red Diamondback Rattlesnake. Notice the characteristic 'pits' of the pit viper

76

Husbandry

Reptiles use the sun for warmth as well as vitamin-D production; therefore, ultraviolet radiation is an important factor in their husbandry. Caution should be used when providing heat and sunlight to reptiles, as overexposure can lead to hyperthermia and burns. Reptile heating lights, pads and rocks are commonly used for heat sources, while UV lights can provide a source of vitamin-D production.

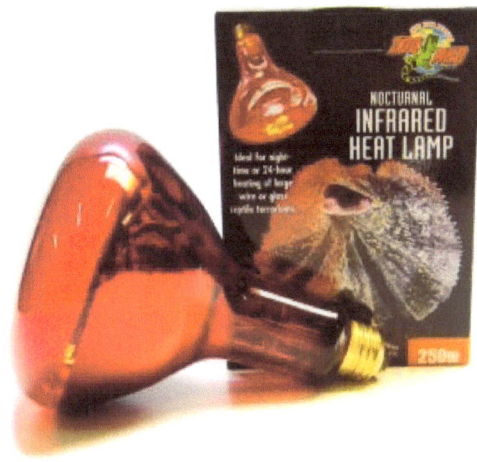

Figure 96: Heat lamps and UV lights are important components to reptile husbandry

Appropriate substrate and plants should be used in terrariums or housing for reptiles. Improper substrate may cause injury to scales or create impactions if swallowed. Some substrates, such as sphagnum moss, can be useful for egg laying material or a source of humidity. Plants should be evaluated for their toxicity; the California Turtle and Tortoise Club maintain a list of poisonous plants. http://www.tortoise.org/general/poisonp.html Water is widely utilized to provide humidity to many species, a source of drinking and an aid in shedding and in egg laying. As with all animals, a source of water should be provided as a minimum standard of animal care.

Feeding

Reptiles are generally placed into two feeding categories: herbivores and carnivores. Most species require regular feeding, but appetite may be variable based on season and ambient temperature. Herbivorous reptiles such as most tortoises and some lizards, require fresh vegetation in the form of leafy greens and kale. Vegetables, like tomatoes and carrots, can be utilized. Some species also will eat flowers such as hibiscus.

Many species of snakes eat rodents such as mice and rats. Immobilization of prey items may be from a venomous bite or constriction. All parts of the prey item are swallowed head-first and digested. Depending on the prey size, swallowing and digestion may take several days; these snake species tend to feed less frequently than others. Some smaller lizards and snakes may consume insects and require more frequent feeding. In all cases, careful observation should be maintained while a live prey animal has been placed in a reptile's cage. It is not uncommon for the prey item to feed on or cause injury to the reptile if left unattended.

Calcium is an important element in the reptilian diet and is generally supplemented to some degree. Always determine the proper dietary requirements for any reptile prior to feeding and caring for them.

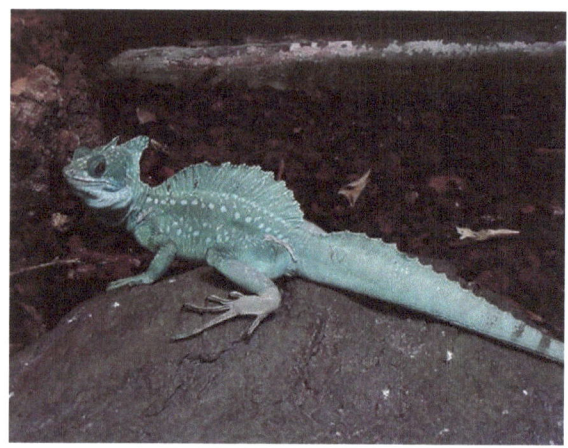

Medical Procedures

Most reptiles are hardy and require little medical care and intervention. Medical procedures may be necessary as a result of conspecific trauma, improper shedding (disectdysis) or reproductive issues.

Wounds to the skin of reptiles can be difficult to treat and require long periods of time for healing. Conspecific wounds may result in punctures, abscesses and fractures, while traumatic injuries from cages may involve shell and feet injury. Many species have size or color dimorphism, while others lack differences between the sexes. In these cases, gender identification may be made by determining the cloacal-tail distance using a metal gender probe.

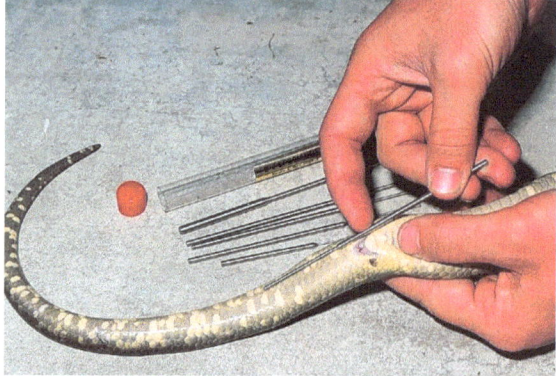

Figure 97: Gender determination using sexing probe depth

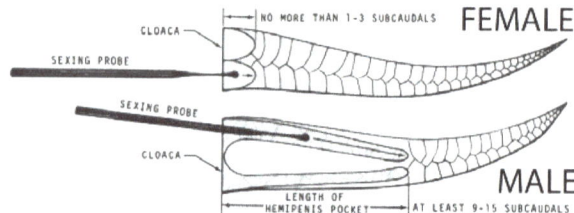

Figure 98: Illustration showing use of sexing probe to determine reptile gender

Laparoscopy can be used to identify internal reproductive structures such as the ovaries or testes. This procedure requires anesthesia and can be minimally invasive.

Dystocia in reptiles can require surgical intervention. Egg binding and a resultant egg yolk coelomitis can lead to surgical removal of eggs.

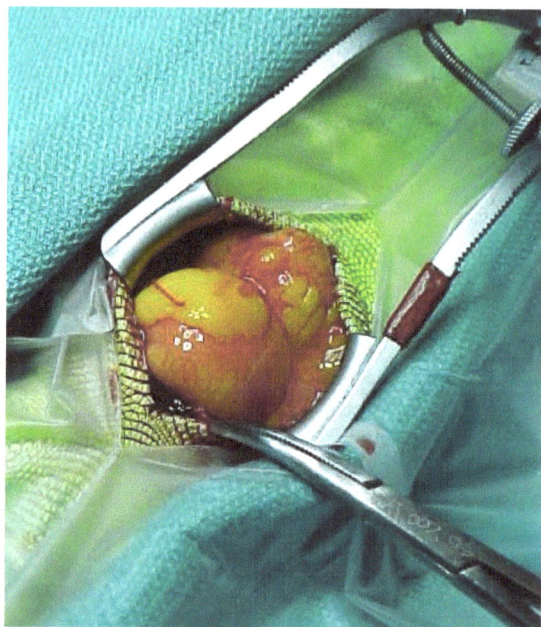

Figure 99: Surgical excision of eggs in an iguana

Wounds can be treated with antiseptic soaps and flushes, as well as cephalosporin antibiotics such as ceftazidime. Sometimes antibiotic beads can be used directly in the wound for long term antimicrobial activity. Antibiotic beads are slowly dissolved and absorbed into the wound site and bloodstream.

78

Fluid therapy can be used to triage reptiles and is calculated based on patient weight. Crystalloid fluids such as, Lactated Ringers, may be given to rehydrate patients or treat anorexia or hypovolemia.

Blood collection is an important diagnostic tool in reptile medicine. As with most animals, it is estimated that ten percent of the patient's blood volume can safely be taken; this equates to roughly one percent of patient's bodyweight, where 1 gram equals one milliliter of blood. One of the easiest locations for blood collection in snakes and lizards is the ventral coccygeal or tail vein. This vessel runs just beneath the coccygeal vertebrae of the tail and is relatively easy to access. A lateral approach can be made on this vessel as well; this may be the preferred method in some species such as crocodilians and other laterally flattened tailed individuals.

Other blood sampling locations include the cephalic and brachial veins as well as the jugular veins. Cardiac venipuncture can be used but is generally reserved as a last resort. Turtles and tortoises have a vascular plexus behind their heads and under the carapace. Often referred to as the sub-carapacial plexus, this area can be used for blood collection. Lymphatic contamination can be a problem in some sites, including the sub-carapacial plexus, so proper interpretation of blood test results should include information about lymph contamination.

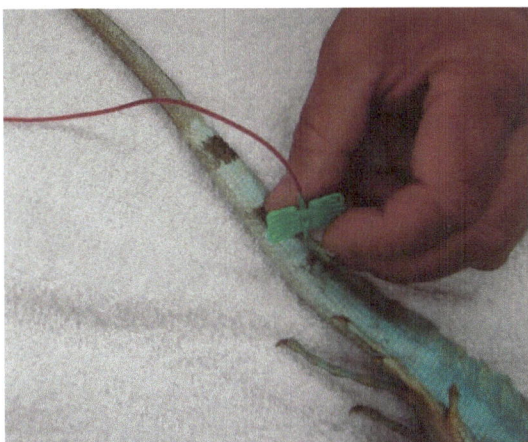

Figure 100: Phlebotomy of the lateral tail vein

Intraosseous catheters (IO catheters) can be used when venous access is limited or unobtainable. IO catheters are driven through the epiphysis of one of the long bones and secured in the lumen of the bone. Fluids are delivered and absorbed by the marrow.

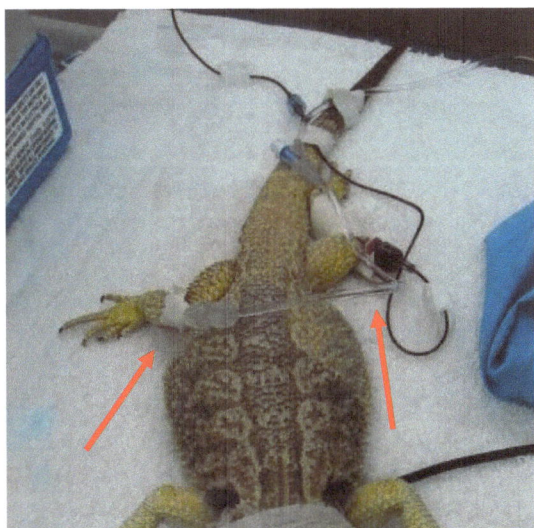

Figure 101: Intraosseous catheters in both tibias of a Bearded Dragon

Anesthesia

Injectable and inhalation type anesthetics can be used in most reptiles. Recently, reversible drugs such as medetomidine have been used because of their ability to be antagonized. Other injectable anesthetics used in reptiles include ketamine and Propofol. Desflurane, a fluorinated anesthetic gas, is commonly used in reptiles because of its improved induction and recovery times. This is based on Desflurane's low solubility coefficient, allowing anesthetic blood/gas levels to be nearly identical. Unfortunately, Desflurane is very expensive and requires a special precision vaporizer, making it less popular to some veterinary practices. As with all anesthetic, overdosing can be a significant problem in reptiles; this is compounded by low patient metabolism and lower body temperatures. Careful patient monitoring should include the observation of spontaneous respiration, heart rate and strength using a Doppler ultrasound unit, as well as patient reflexes, movements and changes in patient coloration. Changes in any of these parameters may suggest excessive anesthetic depth and a precursor to overdosing. A Doppler ultrasound unit, similar to the instrumentation used to hear fetal heartbeats, is very useful in determining heart rates and strength.

Most reptiles should be intubated during anesthesia so that positive pressure ventilation can be performed in the absence of spontaneous breathing. Cole and Cook tubes used for birds are also appropriate for reptiles. Reptiles lack an epiglottis; however, many have strong glottal muscles making intubation more challenging. A spatula can be used as a mouth gag; this can also serve to cover sharp teeth and fangs in venomous species during intubation.

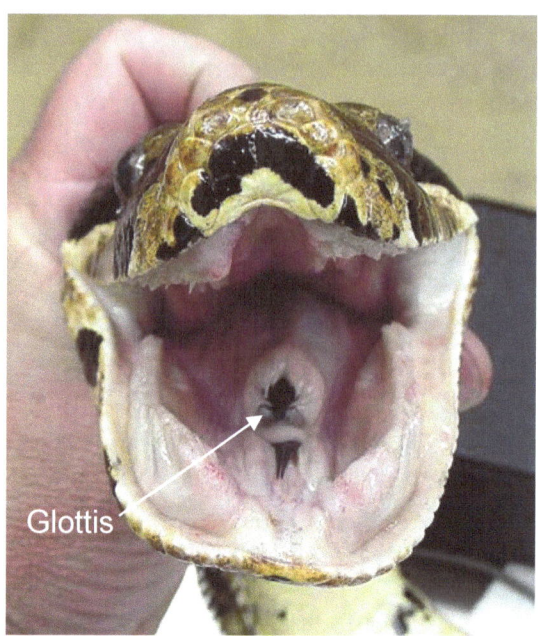

Figure 102: Reptile oropharanyx

Due to reptile physiology, mechanical ventilation may be necessary and beneficial. Respiration rates may not exceed two to four breaths per minute, and in many cases, respiratory quality may be poor. As with birds, periodic mechanical ventilation may insure endotracheal tube patency in the reptile.

Diseases

It is generally assumed that all reptiles carry and potentially transmit the zoonotic disease, Salmonella. For this reason, good hygiene practices should be used when handling reptiles. Ideally, anyone handling reptiles should wear latex gloves, or minimally, wash their hands immediately after working with them. Salmonella is excreted in the feces of reptiles, so care should be taken during routine husbandry practices such as cage cleaning.

Metabolic bone disease causes abnormalities of bones in reptiles and is usually associated with dietary mineral deficiencies or improper exposure to sunlight. Minerals such as calcium, magnesium and phosphorus are important in bone development and density. Vitamin D, acquired by ultraviolet radiation via sunlight, is also an important factor in bone health.

Egg stasis results in the impaction of eggs prior to parturition and can cause discomfort and coelomic infection called peritonitis. The term 'gravid' is used to describe an egg bearing reptile. Egg stasis in a gravid reptile may require surgical intervention if the eggs are not passed in a timely manner. The use of oxytocin, to induce uterine contractions, as well as dinoprostone (Prepidil), a cervical dilator, is sometimes administered prior to surgical intervention.

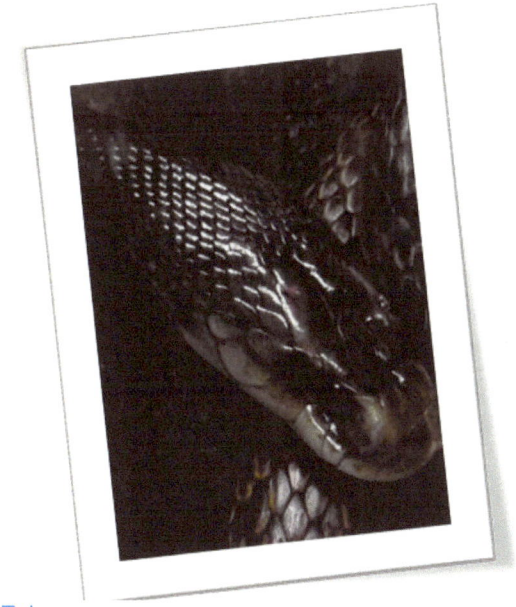
Taipan

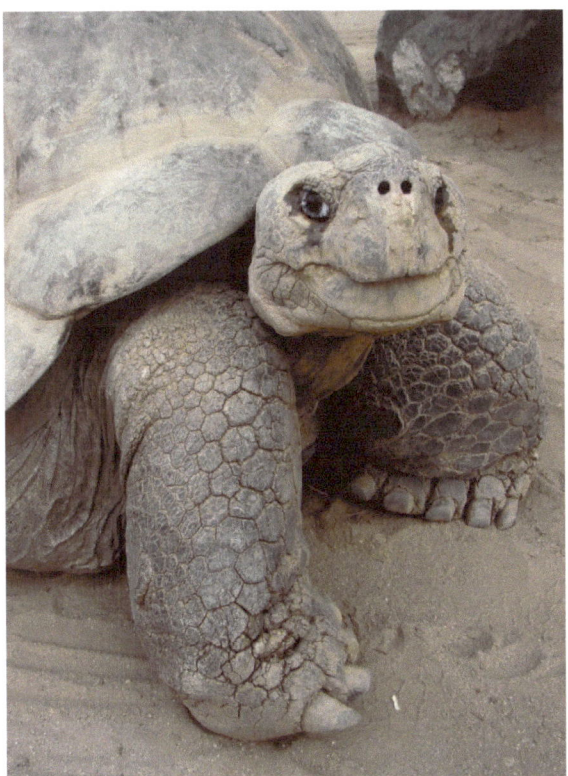
Figure 103: Galapagos Tortoise

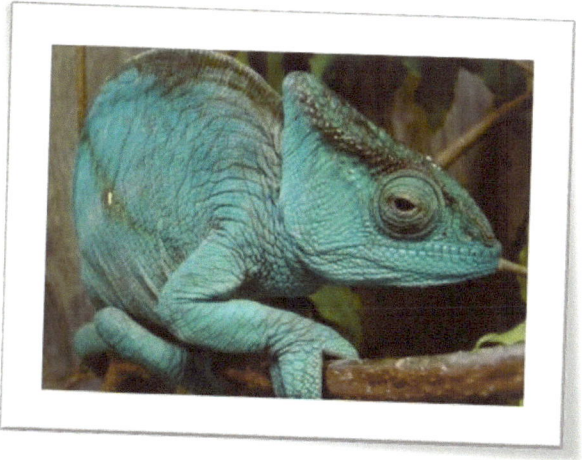
Parson's Chameleon

Nonhuman Primates

Working with nonhuman primates may be limited to those employed at a zoo, research facility, or a caretaker of a rehabilitation facility or sanctuary. Nonhuman primates include old world and new world monkeys and apes, as well as prosimians, such as lemurs, found exclusively on the island of Madagascar. Specifically, the term 'nonhuman primate' means all nonhuman members of the order Primates, including, but not limited to, animals commonly known as monkeys, chimpanzees, orangutans, gorillas, gibbons, apes, baboons, marmosets, tamarins, lemurs, and lorises.

Classification

Primates are generally classified by their geographical origins and phenotypic characteristics. For example, all monkeys have a tail, and all apes lack one. Additionally, most apes are larger than their monkey cousins. Most old world monkeys and all great apes are characterized as having opposable thumbs, a trait that is lacking in new world primates and prosimians. Many new world monkeys have prehensile tails and flattened noses. Old world primates, those from Africa and Asia, are considered an older lineage of primate and have similar characteristics and disease susceptibilities. New world primates are the result of the radiation of primates from Africa into the Americas, specifically South America. It is believed that old world primates may have 'rafted' to South America several millions of years ago when the two continents were much closer together. There are, however, no indigenous non-human primates in North America or Antarctica.

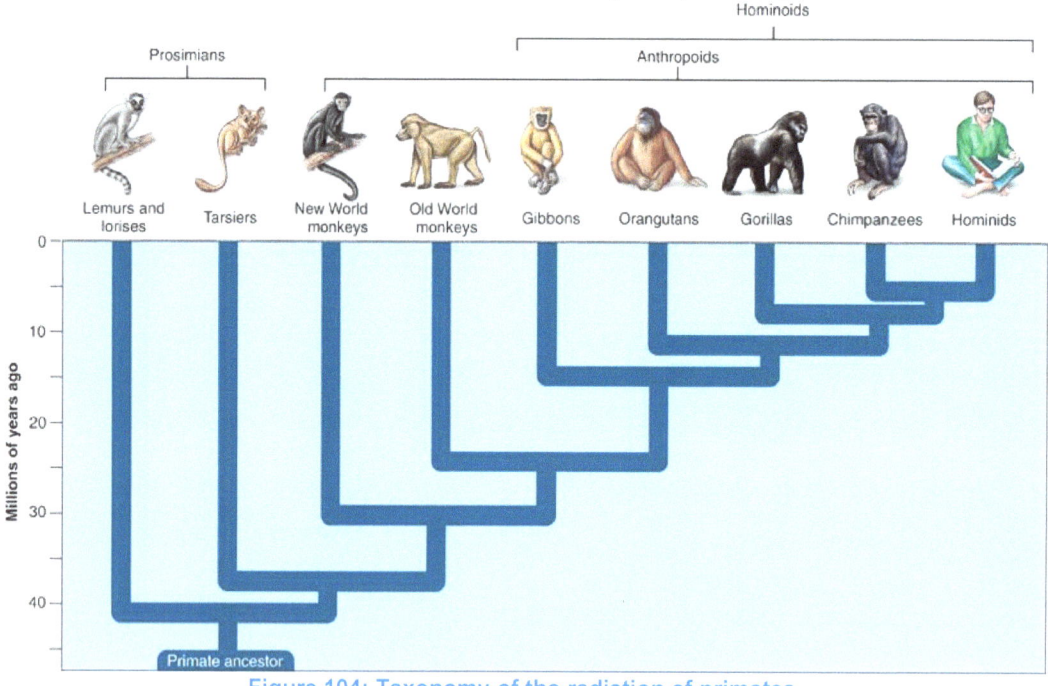

Figure 104: Taxonomy of the radiation of primates

82

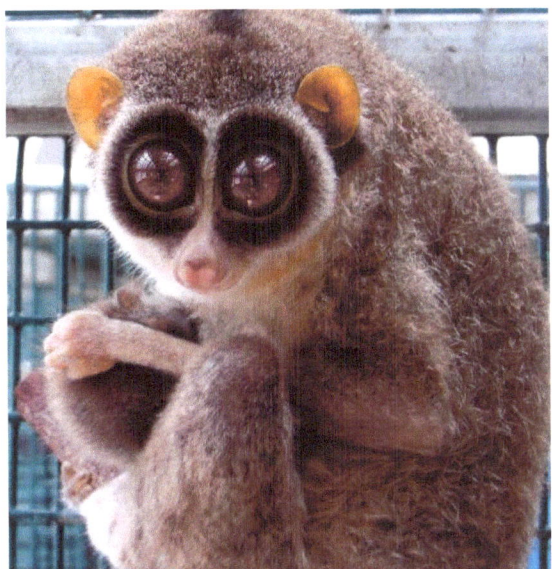
Figure 105: Slender Loris

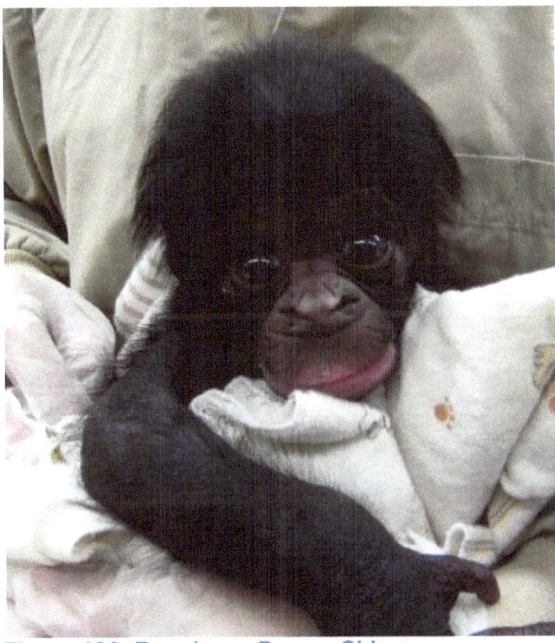
Figure 106: Bonobo or Pygmy Chimpanzee

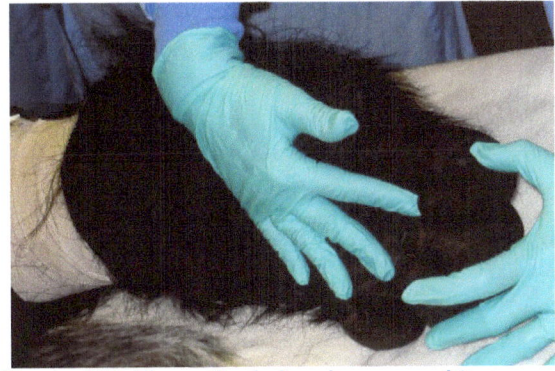
Figure 107: The author's hand compared to a Western Gorilla hand

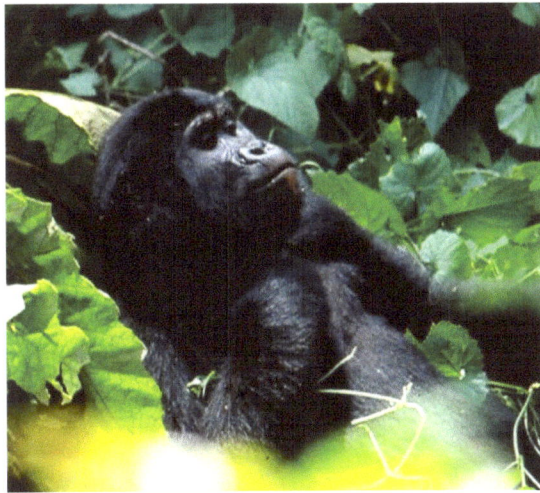
Figure 108: Mountain Gorilla

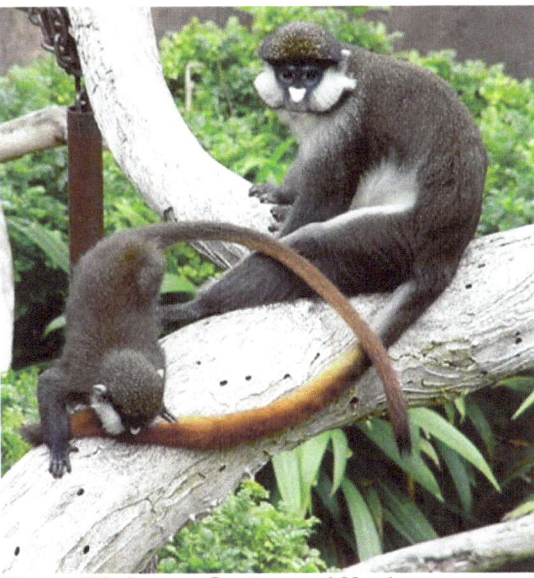
Figure 109: Lesser Spot-nosed Monkey

Primates as Pets

Primates are some of the most breathtaking and interesting animals; however, they may not be the most ideal pet. Primates are agile, tactile, inquisitive and very strong for their size. It is estimated that a chimpanzee is up to five times stronger than a human. The intellect of an ape is thought to be at the cognitive level of a five year old human. This combination of strength and immaturity can be dangerous. Primates, just as humans, may be intimidated by staring, and may display irritation and teeth displaying when provoked.

83

Husbandry

Most primates in captivity can be found in zoos and sanctuaries; private individuals and research facilities make up a small proportion of captive primates. Primates can be messy, destructive and vocal. They require proper space to remain active and healthy. Husbandry for primates includes supplying proper nutrition, fresh water, climbing structures and providing the availability of sunlight. Without these things, primates may become unhealthy, irritable and destructive. Enclosure considerations should take into account the types of plants and substrates; some plants are toxic, and primates may ingest items that can become obstructed. Wires should be of heavy gauge metal, and spacing should be appropriate; primates may squeeze through very small spaces. In general, careful consideration should be made before housing or caring for primates.

Enrichment

Enrichment has become an important aspect of animal husbandry, especially in zoos. Types of enrichment include boomer balls, ropes, toys as well as food mazes and music. Videos can be used to stimulate animals such as primates. The function of enrichment is to improve the quality of life of captive animals and reduce or prevent stereotypical abhorrent behaviors such as pacing, self mutilation and head rocking. Primates can be offered boxes filled with paper and desirable food items; accessing those prizes takes time and provides stimulation to the animal. Additionally, these items, including the box, are safe, even in the event of ingestion. In large institutions such as zoos, enrichment items are evaluated by animal care specialists and

veterinarians to ensure that the items are appropriate and safe.

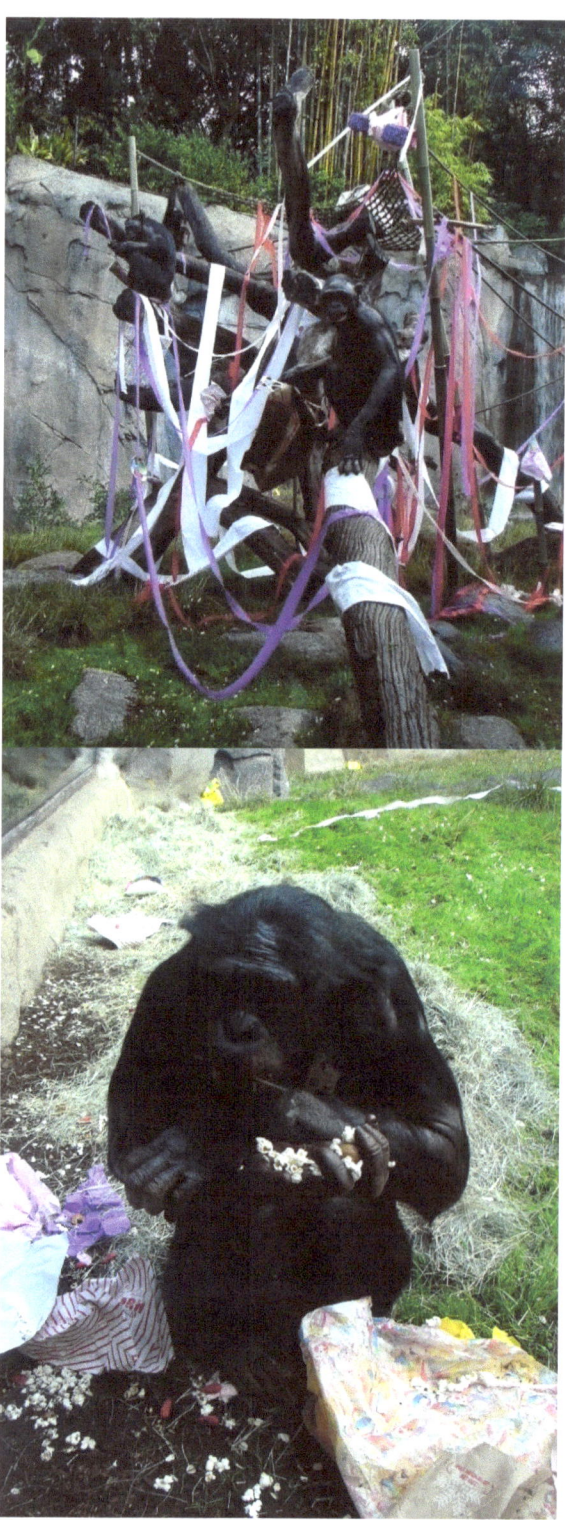

Figure 110: Enrichment for a troop of Bonobos

84

Primates are more cognitive than other species, and are more apt to recognize medications hidden in food items. For this reason, medications are sometimes mixed or inserted into prized food items such as grapes and raisins. It is always more desirable to give oral medications, when possible, as it is less invasive to the patient. Compounding pharmacies have been instrumental in making bitter tasting medications, such as the antibiotic enrofloxacin (Baytril®), taste like grapes or strawberries. They have also increased drug concentrations so less medication must be administered. Electrolyte water is an effective way to provide fluid therapy to a primate if they tolerate drinking. Without patient compliance, medications may have to be delivered by injection.

Vaccinations

Because of the genetic similarity between nonhuman primates and humans, many human vaccines have been used to protect primates against disease. The following vaccinations may be used as a prophylactic measure in primates:

- Rabies vaccine
- Tetanus Toxoid
- Influenza vaccine(great apes)

Ivermectin (Ivomec®), an antiparasitic drug, and tuberculin intradermal skin testing are additional injectable drugs commonly given to primates during routine examination..

Birth Control

Primates, specifically great apes, can be effectively contracepted with common birth control pills used by humans. In zoos, birth control pills are given to female apes to prevent pregnancy while still allowing the maintenance of the social group. Some institutions use melengestrol acetate birth control implants. Commonly known as MGA implants, this slow release drug is surgically inserted under the skin in the interscapular region in primates. MGA implants are easily tolerated once placed, and are able to maintain birth control for about two years. Depot medroxyprogesterone acetate (Depo Provera), a progesterone hormone contraceptive, functions to prevent follicular development and ovulation and can be used in primates. The drug is given intramuscularly every three months to prevent pregnancy.

Other methods of birth control in primates include limiting access of opposite sexes to each other, and to cohabitate only same gender individuals. In some occasions, surgical sterilization is used. In primates, a vasectomy in males, and a hysterectomy in females is performed to preserve gonadal hormones such as testosterone and estrogen produced in the testes and ovaries.

The primary reason for birth control in apes is to prevent over-representation of genetic lines in captive populations. Most captive exotic animals are managed by species survival plans (SSP) in an attempt to maintain a populations' genetic diversity. Housing limitations may play a role in nonhuman primate reproductive management.

Anatomy and Physiology

The anatomy and physiology of primates differs little from dogs, cats, or you. An obvious difference from humans includes the presence of hair covering the entire body and the presence of a tail (monkeys). Other differences, in some, include the following:

- *Gular pouch*
  The presence of a gular or throat pouch, in some species, is part of

the respiratory system and thought to enhance vocalization and communication by individual primates in a forest environment
- *Fermenting stomach*
  Some primates, such as the Vietnamese Douc Langur, are strict herbivorous fermenters like cows and deer
- *Opposable thumbs*
  Present in all great apes and most old world monkeys; absent in most new world monkeys
- *Prehensile tail*
  Found in many new world monkey species and thought to aid in dexterity lost by absence of opposable thumbs

Handling and Restraint

Proper handling and restraining techniques are imperative to ensure the safety of both primates and animal care workers. Due to the strength and potential infectious disease transmission of nonhuman primates, special care and training should be considered prior to working with these animals. With any wild animal, especially primates, secondary containment measures should always be in place to avoid possible escape from a captive situation; even the best animal handlers can lose hold of an animal. For example, when getting a small primate out of a cage, ensure that the cage is in a secure room with no doors left open. Never go into cage holding a primate unless you have prior understanding of that individual. Support if needed, should be available in the event of an unprovoked attack. Always plan for an escape or unrealized threat before it happens.

Protective equipment when handling and interacting with primates may include latex gloves, protective gowns, face masks and eye protection. These items are designed to protect against potential exposure to infectious and zoonotic diseases that may enter the oral and ocular mucosa, as well as through the skin via punctures or open wounds. Some institutions may require the use of N95 particulate masks and face shields when working with high risk primates such as macaques that may carry the simian herpes virus.

Manual Restraint

Manual restraint of primates should be limited to very small species or moribund individuals. The use of appropriate sized nets or towels is an effective means of capture. Once contained in a net or towel, careful securing of the head and body can take place. Gauntlet gloves are essential to prevent unintended biting, however their use can reduce one's dexterity. Manual restraint in a towel or net may be a precursor to anesthetic induction or injection of medication.

Behavioral Restraint

Efforts to do medical procedures on primates without the use of anesthetics have led to tremendous strides in behavioral restraint and manipulation. Animals are trained to present limbs and body regions for examination, sample collection, medication administration, heart and lung auscultation and dental evaluation. The behaviors are trained as part of a daily routine, therefore, desensitizing animals to the procedure or process. This is especially useful for diabetic patients, or for animals that require anesthesia; injections can easily be given without need for the stress of darting or capture. Primates may be more receptive to doing behaviors for their primary caretakers; in many cases, veterinary staff relies on these individuals to inject primates with anesthetic induction drugs.

Chemical Restraint

Ultimately, safely working on a primate requires the use of anesthesia. Large monkeys and apes are incredibly strong, and when under anesthesia, can still be intimidating. Anesthetics are very effective on primates; they require nominal amounts of drugs, and are effectively maintained on gas anesthetics such as isoflurane. Common injectable anesthetics include ketamine, diazepam, midazolam and propofol.

Methods for injecting primates include manual and behavioral methods, as well as restraint devices such as squeeze crates. 'Squeezes' reduce the area in which an animal has in a crate. The back wall of the crate can be pulled towards the front wall, generally made of a perforated metal fence. This immobilizes the animal, allowing for the administration of injectable medications. One of the biggest challenges with squeezes is the resistance from the primate in allowing the wall to close. Additionally, in some cases it is difficult to get the primate into the squeeze.

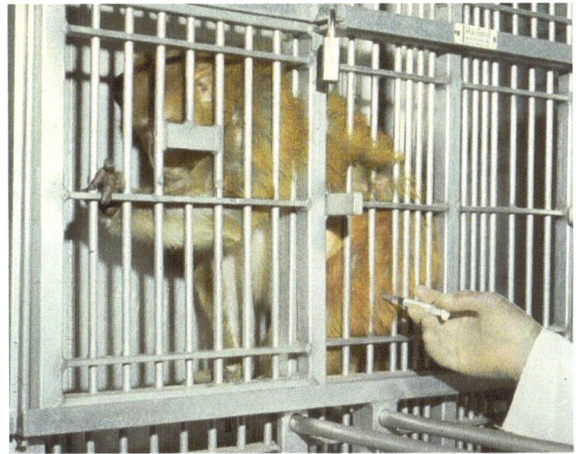

Figure 111: Primate squeeze cage; the rear wall moves toward the front

Wildlife officials and zoo staff, make use of remote injection systems in order to immobilize wild or captive animals that cannot be restrained by other methods. The remote darting system uses charged darts fired by air driven rifles. Much like paintball guns, darts are shot up to one hundred feet at animal targets. Dart flight is affected by wind and gravity, and therefore, practice shots should be made before darting an animal. Most darts are aimed at large muscle bodies of the arm, shoulder, leg and neck in large animals. Primates are generally darted in the quadriceps muscles of the legs; however, due to their speed and agility, an accurate shot can be difficult. Once darted, primates tend to quickly remove the dart; some may chew or otherwise damage it. Once darted, anesthetic induction may take several minutes; primates that climb into trees may fall to the ground when induction proceeds.

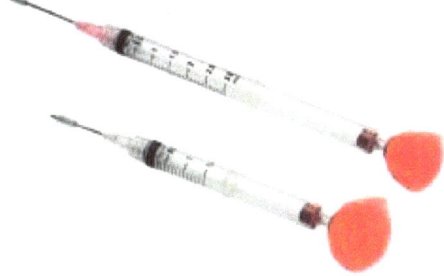

Figure 112: Remote injection darts

Identification

Some primates can be identified by color differences or behaviors, while others show size dimorphism. In general, male primates tend to be larger than females, and if colored, the males are generally more vibrant. Primates have external genitalia, making determination of gender plausible. Some female apes exhibit enormous vulvas during estrus. Primate caretakers may identify individual animals by behavioral characteristics, such as aggression, shyness, dominance or sexual gestures, while others may be vocal, playful or sit in a particular area consistently.

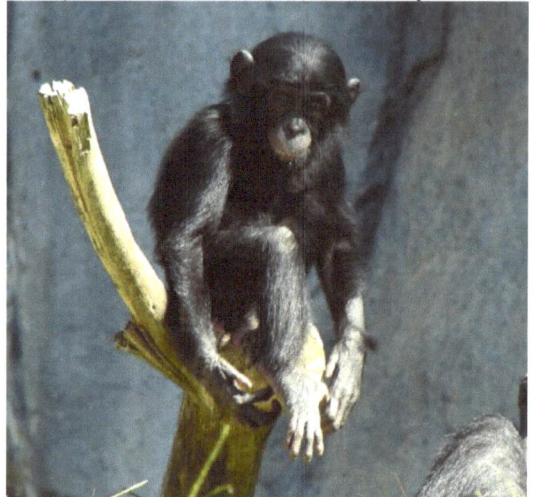
Figure 113: Juvenile Bonobo sitting on tree limb

Permanent forms of identification are very important for tracking individuals that may be part of a breeding colony, a species survival plan (SSP), or for trafficking documentation if moved to other institutions or states. The most common forms of identification include the microchip and tattoo.

The microchip is a small rice-sized implant that is placed under the skin in animals; usually in the interscapular region. The chip is delivered inside a 12ga needle; once under the skin, the plunger ejects the chip from the needle. A special microchip reader is used to scan the identification number in the chip. Most readers must be waved over the chip to get a reading. Some companies claim to have readers that can pick up the chip at a distance of several feet. The benefit of this is being able to read a chip with the animal at a distance. The reader is not effective through metal caging or bars, but works well through plastic and plywood crates. The microchip has no battery, and therefore is thought to last the life of the animal. A typical microchip number may

contain a series of numbers and letters, similar to a license plate. In some cases, such as with bears, microchips are placed in the animals' lip. Due to the food driven behavior of bears, they will often come up to the cage when offered food; the animal can easily be scanned at that time. Some primates are trained to present their chest and back; this makes microchip reading in the interscapulary area accomplishable. Tattoos have been used prior to the advent of microchips, and are still used in some cases. Tattooing equipment for animals is the same that is used in people. Due to the painful nature of the procedure, tattooing is usually done while the animal is anesthetized. In primates, tattoos are frequently placed on the inner thigh or under the upper lip. Most species have lighter skin in the inner limbs, and most have pink oral mucus membranes. Even with dark skinned animals, tattoos can be visible. Prior to placing a tattoo, the area is shaved with a number 40 clipper blade. A light coating of petroleum jelly serves to reduce ink 'bleeding' during tattooing. Tattoos are normally numerical, such as accession numbers or other identifiers for the individual. Names are generally not used for tattoos.

Anesthesia
Once injected or gas anesthetized, most primates do well under anesthesia. During induction, however, close attention should be kept on respiration rate and quality; it is advisable to place primates in an inclined position, when possible, to reduce the complications of aspiration and dyspnea. A foam wedge or rolled up towel serve to provide inclination when placed in the axilla of primates during anesthetic induction. Primates are well maintained for long

procedures with isoflurane gas anesthesia.

Once at an appropriate anesthetic level, primates should be intubated in order to maintain a patent airway. Primates, unlike most animals, have a prominent laryngospasm; this reflex of the larynx is caused by stimulation of the endotracheal tubes. The application of topical lidocaine reduces the effects of laryngospasm, and enables tracheal intubation. Primates have a relatively short tracheal inlet when compared with most species. It is important to measure endotracheal distance prior to intubation and determine proper placement after tube placement. If an endotracheal tube is passed beyond the carina, or tracheal bifurcation, bronchial collapse will occur in the non-intubated lung lobe.

Ausculting the lungs for air sounds is a standard practice to determine proper endotracheal tube placement. Once placed, the endotracheal tube should be tied in behind the head; most primates lack long canine teeth and snout that enable the securing of the tube in this location. A rubber band may be used as a securing mechanism for small primates. Some very small primates such as Loris' and marmosets' may benefit from a Cole tube for intubation as traditional cuffed tubes may be too large.

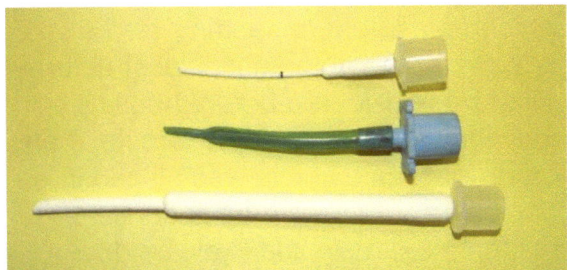
Figure 114: Cole and Cook endotracheal tubes

Due to primates sometimes dark skin color, pulse oximetry may be difficult to assess. Good readings may be obtained

from the cheek in most species, the tongue, however, tends to be small compared to other species, and placement may be difficult. In addition, salivation may cause oximeter movement when placed on the tongue; gauze placed on the tongue may counter this affect. Other locations for pulse oximetry readings include the digits, penis, scrotum and vulva. These areas seem to be less pigmented, even in dark skinned species.

Indirect blood pressure readings can be easily obtained from the limbs or tail. Fur thickness may cause variations from true blood pressure values, so pressure trends may be more useful than absolute numbers. Direct blood pressure readings are usually obtained from the femoral artery, as other arteries may be quite small in some species. Intravenous catheter placement is a prudent standard of care with primates for the following reasons:

- Venus access allows for quick and easy anesthetic adjustments for patients that are rousing.
- Venus access is essential for anesthetic emergencies
- Blood sampling and intra-operative blood chemistries can be easily obtained via IV catheters.

The posterior saphenous vein is an exceptional site for IV catheterization in primates. This robust vessel is easily accessible and tends to be more tolerable than a traditional cephalic vein catheter. In apes, the cephalic vein is a good alternative to the posterior saphenous, as these animals generally have large forearm vascularity. Short term IV catheters can be secured with tape, staples or sutures, whereas long term catheters should be bandaged well. Bandaging of the whole leg in primates is an effective way to reduce catheter manipulation by the patient. Covering the IV line with tape may reduce the incidence of punctures from chewing and biting.

Phlebotomy is achievable from the femoral, cephalic, cubital or posterior saphenous veins. The cubital vein, located in the crux of the medial elbow, is the same vessel that samples are acquired from humans. The femoral veins will yield the greatest volume of blood for collection, as the smaller peripheral veins tend to collapse with overzealous syringe aspiration. Due to the infectious disease potential, the use of a vacutainer system for blood collection is optimal. Vacutainers allow blood to be collected directly from the needle to the blood tube, therefore, eliminating the need for a syringe. Additionally, using butterfly catheters for venipuncture, in conjunction with a vacutainer, allows for movement during blood tube swapping. Using a syringe for blood collection requires the needle to be removed from the patient and inserted into the blood tube; this increases the chance of blood cell destruction and potential for the accidental blood exposure by a needle stick.

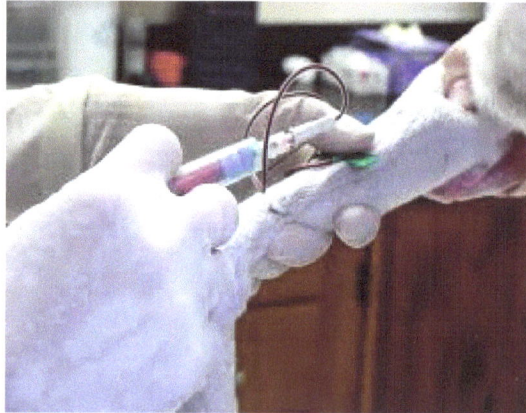

Figure 115: The use of a butterfly catheter and vacutainer for blood collection

Recovery is one of the most crucial times for anesthetic procedures. Just as with induction, primates benefit from an inclined position during recovery. This position reduces the potential for aspiration as well as improves respiratory efficiency. Extubation should occur when pharyngeal reflexes are strong. During this time, the patient can be safely secured with its arms behind its back, or if large, can be rested on its arm in a secure crate.

Reproduction and Breeding

Unlike solitary animals, primates, including humans, tend to be very social in nature. The social group structure is variable depending on the species, but may be of one of the following types:

- *Monogamous family groups-* paired individuals and their offspring
- *Polygynous groups-*one male and many females
- *Polyandrous groups-*several males breeding with one female
- *Multi-male multi-female groups-* no monogamous bond, males and females have a variety of mates
- *Single female and her offspring-* male is solitary except for mating
- *Fission/fusion individuals-* individuals enter and leave the group periodically

This means, that depending on the species of the primate, social structures must be considered before housing individuals together. For example, if an unfamiliar male gorilla was placed in an enclosure with a silverback gorilla and his females, he would likely be driven off, exiled or killed by the dominant silverback.

90

Though many primate groups or troops contain a strong dominant male, many species are matriarchal; females make most decisions for the troop. Sexual receptivity, mate selection and mating are generally established by the females in the troop. Sex is linked to the females 'estrus' cycle. Pheromones, vulvar swelling, color changes, and 'presenting' are indicators of sexual receptivity by females.

Most primates have a single birth followed by a significant parental investment when compared to other animals. Males tend to be providers of food and protection during natal development. Some females in the troop have been known to foster unwanted babies from inexperienced or uninterested mothers.

In general, the function of sex is that of procreation and gene preservation. Bonobos or pygmy chimpanzees, however, use sex for non-procreative purposes. For bonobos, sex is used as a means of conflict resolution, dominance or female/female bonding. Instead of violence, bonobos will resolve issues with individuals in the troop with heterosexual sex, digital probing and sodomy. Masturbation is not uncommon for male primates kept in captivity.

The reproductive anatomy of nonhuman primates consists of external genitalia including the penis and scrotum in the male, and vulva in the female. Genitalia are colorful in some species and others like the male howler monkey of Central America, have a large white pendulous scrotal sack. Vulvar enlargement coincides with estrus in most species; however, bonobo females have overtly large vulvas that do not change size. Little menstrual bleeding occurs during estrus in most species. The menstrual cycle of most non-human primates is similar to humans, usually twenty-five to thirty-five days.

Diseases

Primates bring with them the concern of infectious disease transmission due to their close genetic relationship with humans. Infectious diseases, such as the common cold, may have significant impacts on primates and their troops. Other infectious diseases of concern when working with primates include salmonella, campylobacter, tuberculosis, Ebola and simian herpes virus. Animal care staff should make efforts to eliminate exposures to primate bodily fluids. Blood, urine, saliva and other bodily excretions can transmit infectious diseases. Likewise, caretakers of primates should minimize contact when working with these species and experiencing cold or flu symptoms, as primates can be susceptible to human pathogens.

Disease	Type	Transmission	Zoonotic
Tuberculosis	Bacterial	Airborne	Yes
Ebola	Viral	Bodily fluids	Yes
Simian Herpes	Viral	Bodily fluids	Yes
Salmonella	Bacterial	Feces	Yes
Campylobacter	Bacterial	Feces	Yes

Table 28: Primate diseases

91

Nutrition

Primates eat a variety of food items. Most are herbivorous and eat fruits and vegetables. Processed foods such as extruded pellets and biscuits can provide essential nutrients when offered in conjunction with natural browse. Some primates are specialized fermenters of specific leaves and branches; these animals can be difficult to maintain in captivity due to their special dietary requirements. Even though most primates are vegetarians, some, like baboons, have been known to eat animal protein when it is available and easily accessible. Baboons have been seen feeding on flamingo flocks in Africa; this is a seasonal exploit and is not a typical dietary item.

Positive reinforcement can be fortified with the use of food. Food 'rewards' that may be highly coveted by primates include peanuts, grapes, raisins, melon and nectar. Although these items may not constitute a balanced diet, their use has enabled amazing behavioral training in primates.

Vital Statistics

Nonhuman primates have physiological properties similar to other animals. As expected, smaller primates will have higher resting heart rates and respiratory rates than larger primates. Blood pressure values are consistent with most species, including humans, and would be expected to be around an ideal systolic pressure of 120mmHg and diastolic of 80mmHg (mmHg stands for millimeters of mercury, the unit of measure for blood pressure). Primates have an internal body temperature of approximately 98.2 degrees Fahrenheit.

Species	Example	Size(average)	Longevity
Prosimians			
Lemurs	Ring-tailed lemur, Sifaka, Aye Aye	30g to 10kg	20-30 years
Loris'	Slender loris, Slow loris, Pygmy loris, Galago	100g to 1kg	12-15 years
New World Primates			
Marmosets	Pygmy Marmoset, Goeldi's Marmoset, Moustached Tamarin	120g to 15kg	6-15 years
Monkeys	Capuchin, Howler monkey,	2-10kg	15-45years
Old World Primates			
Monkeys	Spot-nosed monkey, Baboon, Lion-tailed Macaque, Mandrill, Colobus monkey, Vervet monkey	700g-50kg	15-30 years
Lesser Apes	Siamang, Gibbon	10-14kg	25-40 years
Apes	Chimpanzee, Bonobo	30-65kg	50 years
	Gorilla	140-200kg	35-50 years
	Sumatran Orangutan	30-150kg	40-60 years

Table 29: Prosimians, New World and Old World primates and vital statistics

Holistic Medicine

Holistic medicine, sometimes called complimentary medicine, uses alternative therapies to treat ailments. Holistic medicine, derived from the word 'whole', looks at health and disease from a mental, spiritual, and physical basis; it looks at the whole body, not just the disease. It is humane, gentle, and minimally invasive and focuses on the patient's well-being. Conventional medicine, by contrast, uses medications and surgery to treat disease. Pet owners may opt for 'alternative' medicine when conventional medicine proves to be ineffective or has side effects.

Let's compare:
A person, who is stressed, has a poor diet, and gets little sleep, may suffer from insomnia and depression.

- The conventional medicine approach may be to prescribe anti-depressants and sleeping pills
- The holistic approach might be to work out ways to improve the person's sleep and diet

The holistic veterinarian is interested in nutrition, family relationships, hygiene, and stress factors that may be the basis for the ailment. The aim of the holistic veterinarian is to ascertain the reason for the symptoms and determine why the body has become so imbalanced. He or she seeks to promote the animal's natural healing processes and energy and tries to use the least toxic, least invasive, and most nurturing path to healing.

Types of Holistic Medicine

Massage
- Stimulates the lymphatic system
- Eliminates toxins and promotes healing
- Improves the pet's disposition
- Improves their circulation
- Increases their range of motion
- Can help to prevent injury
- Reduces inflammation
- Relieves tension

Hydrotherapy
- Hydrotherapy treatments are performed in a water filled tub
- Improves fitness and muscle tone with resistance effect of water
- Thermal effects
- Produces hydrostatic pressure for treatment of edema
- Useful in weak patients and those with compromised joints
- Useful in the treatment of arthritis, fractures and central nervous system disorders

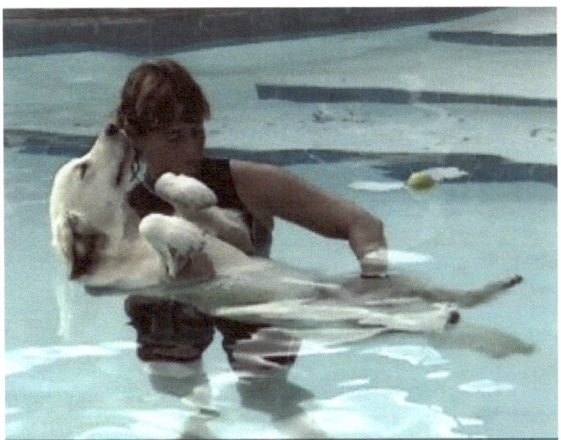
Figure 116: Physical therapy in a pool

Acupuncture

- Fundamentals of acupuncture are based on the Chinese principle of QI (chee) or 'life energy'
- Needles are placed under the skin in specific energy points and channels called meridians
- Stimulation of energy points corrects imbalances in the flow of QI
- Response to acupuncture is generally seen after several treatments
- Used to treat variety of disorders

Chiropractic

- Joint manipulations, also called adjustments, are designed to realign the spine, joints, and the body as a whole
- Causes changes in animal's attitude and performance
- Signs of stiffness, soreness, muscle spasms are indicators of the body's misalignment

Herbal Medicine

- Homeopathy is a system of alternative medicine based on the doctrine that 'like cures like' suggesting a substance that causes the symptoms of a disease in healthy people will cure similar symptoms in sick people
- The natural pharmaceutical science that uses various plants, minerals and vitamins in very small doses to stimulate the body's natural defenses
  - Nutraceuticals
- Giving small doses that cause symptoms such as allergy injections

- No clear scientific explanation and little scientific research
- No FDA monitoring

Aromatherapy

- The art and science of using essential oils from plant sources for the health and well-being of the patient
- Aromatherapy uses the life force of plants and affect the patient on both mental and emotional planes
- Oils are inhaled and stimulate the olfactory nerve
- This quick acting therapy sends messages to limbic area of the brain which is responsible for memory, learning and emotion

Other Therapies

- Gold beads are inserted under the skin at specific locations and are used to provide long term acupuncture point stimulation
- Magnets and magnetic collars are said to increases blood flow, analgesia, and cell growth
- Lasers are used for their anti-inflammatory and analgesic properties

Reproduction

Reproduction in most species is the process of procreating offspring from parent individuals. Reproduction is hormonally driven, although, other factors such as photoperiod (length of daylight) and environmental temperature may play a role in some species. The process of sexual reproduction creates gene mixing between parent individuals; whereas, asexual reproduction generates identical copies of parent genes, and thus, less genetic diversity. The fetal reproductive anatomy in both sexes is very similar until hormones and sex chromosomes drive the production of gender specific structures. For example, in the presence of estrogen, the fetal gamete producing structures become the ovaries; whereas, in the presence of testosterone, they become the testes.

General Female Anatomy

The general female reproductive anatomy in mammals is similar in most species; most structures are internalized.

The internal structures include the vagina, cervix, uterus, uterine horns and ovaries. In species that produce multiple offspring, the uterine horns are elongated, which enables the implantation of multiple fertilized eggs. The vulva is the external reproductive structure in the female. In some species a prominent clitoris is present. Most species show vulvar enlargement, some quite profound, during estrus and sexual receptivity. The reproductive anatomy of female birds' is all internalized, with a well developed ovary and oviduct present. The reproductive system of the female bird terminates at the cloaca.

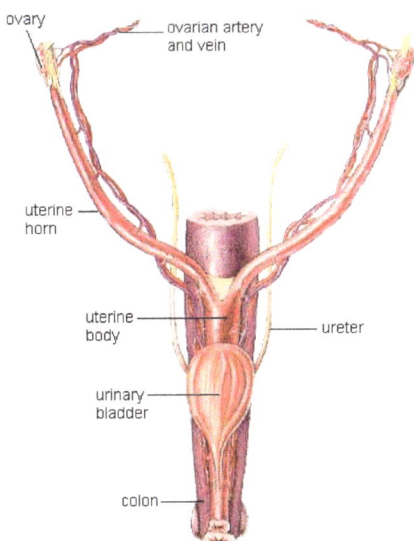

Figure 117: General female reproductive anatomy

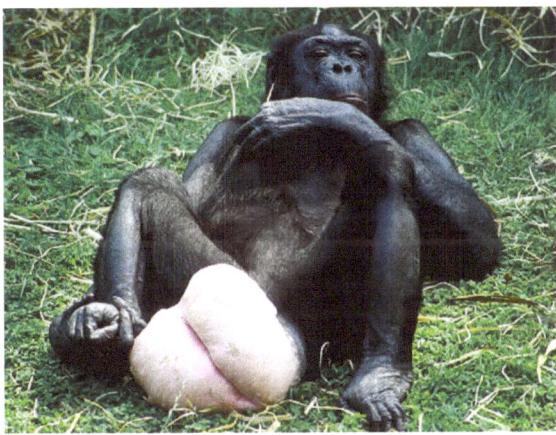

Figure 118: Female Bonobo with vulvar enlargement

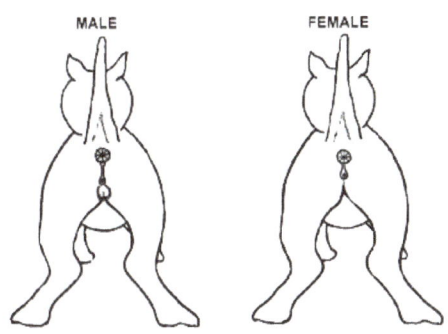

Figure 119: Most genders can be distinguished by anal-genital distance

The Estrus Cycle

The estrus cycle is variable in most mammals. Commonly called 'heat', estrus is a hormonally driven process. The process of estrus in mammals does the following:

- Cause the formation and release of a gamete (egg) from the ovaries
- Prepare the endometrial lining for egg implantation and nourishment
- Stimulate sexual receptivity
- Clear the endometrium if egg implantation does not occur

Most animals clear the endometrium by its reabsorption into the body. Some, like dogs and humans, shed this lining in the form of menstruation.

If impregnation occurs, the endometrium will remain and provide vascular nourishment and attachment for the placenta and its developing fetus. Estrus cycling is mediated by the release of an egg, or ovulation, by the female, under the two following circumstances:

- Spontaneous ovulation
  - Ovulation occurs without copulation; usually hormonally driven
- Induced ovulation
  - Ovulation occurs as a result of copulation (coitus) which causes hormone release

Estrus cycling frequency can be described as one of the following:

- Seasonally monoestrous
- Diestrous
- Polyestrous
- Seasonally polyestrous

Species such as bears, foxes and deer have single annually (seasonal monoestrous), predictable estrous cycles.

Diestrous species usually have two estrous cycles per year. Polyestrous species such as cows, cats and pigs, have many estrous cycles per year if they are not impregnated. Seasonally polyestrous species such as horses, sheep and goats, go into estrus cycles repetitively during particular times of the year until bred. These species usually align breeding and parturition with environmental conditions that will lead to abundant food for their offspring. This is an important consideration, as resources are what maintain a species. In years of drought, for example, less herbivore's have food and are produced, and as a result, predatory species may suffer.

Species	Estrus	Frequency
Dog	3 weeks	5-11 months
Cat	14-21 days	Induced
Rabbit		Induced
Horse	21 days	Annually
Cow	21 days	
Pig	18 days	
Guinea Pig	16-18 days	
Gerbil	6-8 days	
Mouse	4-5 days	3 days
Rat	4-5 days	3 days
Hamster	4 days	

Table 30: Estrus cycles in a variety of species

Gestation

Once fertilized and implanted, the developing fetus will rapidly develop. The time from conception to parturition (birth), is often referred to as the gestation. If the date of conception is known, the gestation time for that species can very closely determine the ultimate date of parturition. Gestation can vary by a few days, or with the feline family, can be postponed until circumstances are ideal.

Gestation in birds, more appropriately called incubation, is the time required to hatch an offspring from its egg.

Species	Gestation (days)
Mouse	21
Rat	22
Hamster	33
Cat	62
Dog	65
Pig	115
Sheep	145
Human	259-294
Cow	283
Horse	336
Giraffe	420-450
Rhinoceros	487
Elephant	600-660

Table 31: Gestation periods in a variety of species

General Male Anatomy

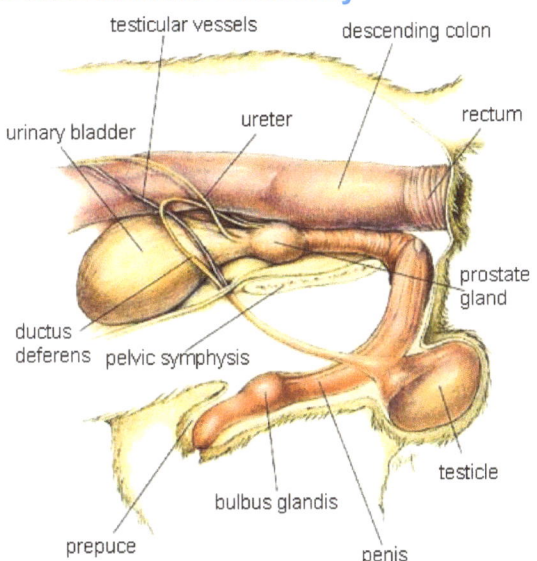

Figure 120: General male reproductive anatomy

Internal Structures
The prostate is located near the bladder and serves to produce the fluid responsible for transporting sperm during copulation. The sperm and fluid together, called semen, travels down the urethra and is ejaculated out of the penis. The urethra also serves to expel

urine from the bladder during urination. Birds lack a true urethra and penis,

External Structures
The external structures of the male mammal include the penis and scrotum which holds the testicles. The reproductive structures of the mammalian mammal are located in the inguinal region of the body. The penis, though usually cranial to the scrotum, resides caudal in marsupials. Many theories exist for this phenomenon, however none have been substantiated. Theories for an external scrotum include temperature regulation and sexual prowess.

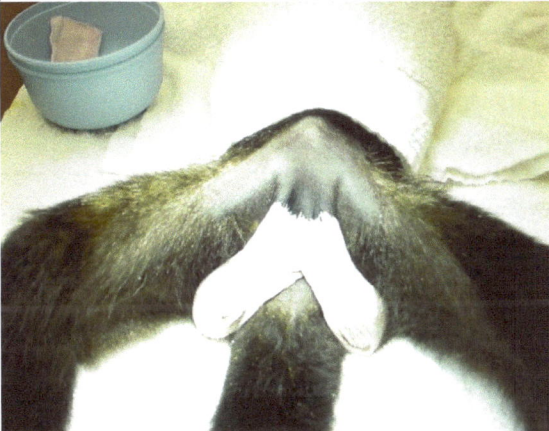

Figure 121: Howler monkey scrotum; penis is cranial to scrotum (under towel)

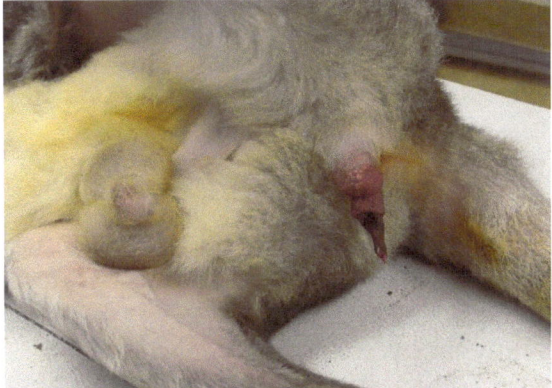

Figure 122: Red kangaroo scrotum; notice penis is behind (caudal) to scrotum

The penis or copulatory organ of the male is usually covered in a protective sheath called the prepuce. The prepuce protects the delicate penile skin from injury and the elements. In some species, a flaccid penis may not be easily visible; this is common in cold climate species. When erect, the mammalian penis can be variable in length and structure. In male koalas, for example, the penis is forked at the distal tip in order to access the females' bifurcated uterus. Others have bulbus glands in the penis that enlarge during copulation. This is commonly referred as being 'tied', as it appears that the breeding pair is connected and unable to be separated. Many species have a penile bone called an os penis. This bone gives rigidity to the penis and aids in entering the females vaginal vault. The scrotum in mammals supports the testicles and is usually externalized. Some species have testicles that can be internalized inguinally, making it difficult to easily determine gender In all species except marsupials, the scrotum is located caudal to the penis. The testicles are the site of male gamete production in the form of sperm.

Birds lack a true penis; however, anseriformes (ducks and geese) and struthioniformes (ostriches and emus) have a penile structure called a phallus.

Process of Intercourse

Intercourse also referred to as coitus or breeding, is the sexual process of transferring genetic material from male to female. In nearly all species, intercourse facilitates procreation and its function is not that of pleasure. In primates, however, intercourse takes on many facets of sexuality, including procreation, dominance, conflict resolution, pleasure and bonding. Intercourse in mammals is preceded by receptivity by the female; if receptive, males mount the female from behind. In

birds, receptivity is usually initiated by pre-breeding displays and courtship by the male. Copulation in birds requires the male to mount the back of the female; to maintain position; the male may grasp or bite the back of the female's neck, a behavior also seen in mammals. In birds, however, the male will rest his feet on the females back as part of copulation.

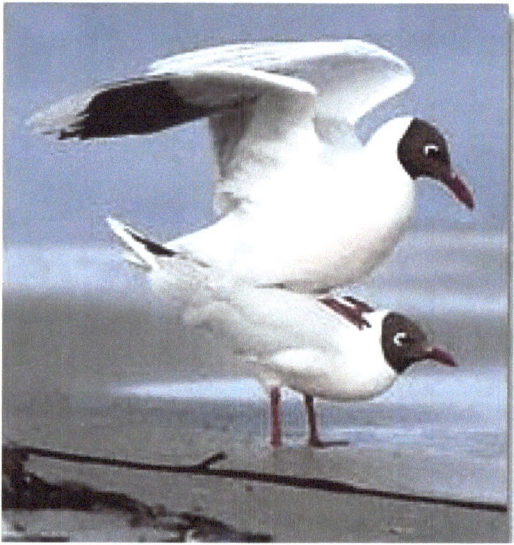
Figure 123: Male birds' sit on the females' back during copulation

Mating Systems

Most birds and a small number of mammal species are monogamous. This type of pair bonding may be seasonal or lifelong. These species are more likely to maintain a territory and share in nest building, incubation and feeding of the offspring.

Other mating strategies used by animals include:

- Polygyny
- Polyandry

Polygyny accounts for a small portion of bird species and most mammal species. In this system, a male mates with many females. This can be commonly seen in herd species like deer and cattle where the male provides protection for the herd. Additionally, the females breed with the strongest male, thus insuring optimal genetic health of their offspring. Polyandry systems are not common to birds or mammals; in this system a female mates with several males. This strategy causes paternity confusion and sperm competition.

Promiscuity may occur by lesser ranking males in a group or by females wishing to mate with an individual other than the dominant male.

Offspring

In general, mammals have a longer and larger investment in childbearing and rearing. Mammals grow at a slower rate than birds, and therefore, parental care is extensive. Gestation is relatively long in mammals, while incubation in birds is relatively short. Once hatched, a golden eagle for example, will be as large as its parents in about two months. A dog, by contrast, is considered full grown at sixteen months of age.

Offspring can be characterized by the magnitude of parental care required after birth or hatching. The following terms describe the offspring types:

- Altricial
- Semi-altricial
- Precocial
- Semi-precocial

Altricial offspring are completely dependent on parent individuals for sustenance, protection, warmth and general care. These individuals are hairless or featherless, with closed eyes. Examples include mice, rats, marsupials and nearly one half of all bird species including songbirds, jays, sparrows and finches.

Semi-altricial species have hair or down feathers, may or may not have open eyes, and are otherwise altricial.

Precocial species are born or hatched with hair or down feathers, and are able to ambulate, leave the nest or den and feed independently. Ducks and geese most ungulates, and guinea pigs are considered precocial.

Semi-precocial species typically stay in the nest or den and are fed by the parents.

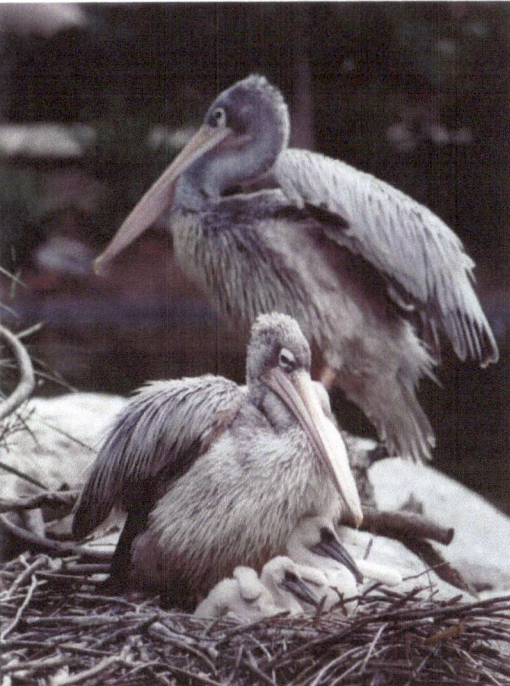

Figure 124: Pink-backed Pelicans with chicks

Common Reproductive Problems

Nutrition, toxins, diseases, can all be factors leading to reproductive problems in animals. Large fetal size or death can lead to surgical intervention in any species. Dystocia, meaning difficult birth, is used to describe a problem with delivery during parturition.

Dystocia in birds may include egg binding; after egg laying there can also be problems with chick hatching. In 1972, DDT, used as a pesticide for decades, was banned in the United States because of its affects on the environment, especially birds. Thin eggshells and the resultant chick death led to the near extinction of the bald eagle and peregrine falcon.

99

Grooming

The Grooming Facility

The grooming facility may be an independent business or a component of a veterinary hospital facility. In addition to grooming, a veterinary practice can accommodate animals that may require sedation for grooming or need additional medical care while being bathed. Some clients have their pets groomed at the end of their pet's boarding stay at the veterinary clinic. Regardless of the locale, a grooming area will have a washing tub for bathing, and an area for drying. Additionally, there will be a variety of grooming products available such as shampoos, dips, combs, brushes and nail trimmers.

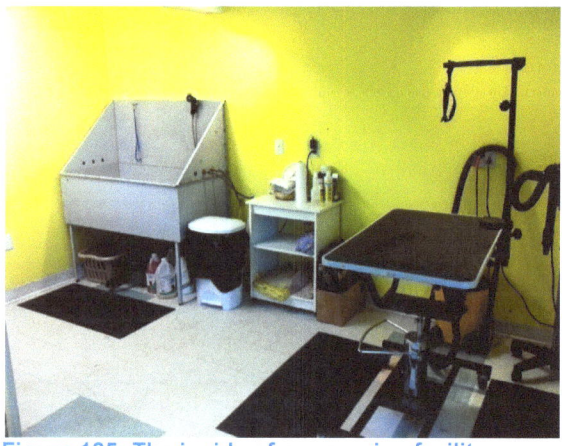

Figure 125: The inside of a grooming facility

Ideally, the bathing tub will be low enough to allow a large pet to enter without being lifted, and be ergonomically friendly for the grooming staff to work comfortably. A ceramic household bathtub may be used, however, care must be taken when lifting heavy animals into it. A non-slip mat may be beneficial when placing a pet on the slippery surface of the tub.

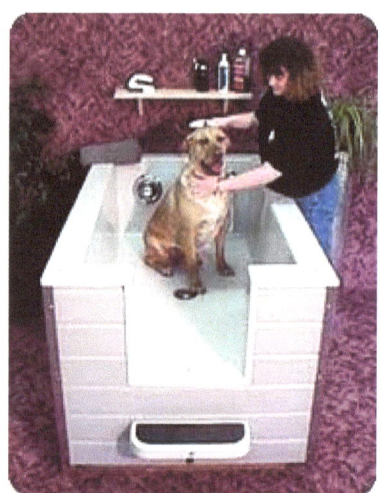

Figure 126: Bathing tub

Heat lamps can be beneficial and dangerous when used as a means to dry a bathed animal. Care must be taken not to place the lamp too close to the pet, or enable them access to any electrical wiring coming from the light source. In general, when using a heat lamp, ensure that the pet can move away from the heat source. Personnel should check on animals frequently.

A heat dryer, when used properly, much like a blow dryer used at home, is a safe way to dry your pet. Warm air flowing through the pet's kennel after being bathed, speeds up the drying process considerably compared to heat lamps. Care should be taken to keep all electrical wiring away from the pet's reach.

Get assistance when lifting heavy animals into a bathing tub

Shampoos

Shampoos are selected by the needs of the pet and the desires of the client. Some shampoos are specially designed for sensitive skin, or may provide flea control. Most are pH balanced for animals, therefore, shampoos made for people may not be appropriate. A good shampoo will not produce a lot of suds when lathered, and therefore will rinse easily. In general, pet shampoos are designed to clean, condition and contain a fragrance to improve the scent of your pet.

When choosing a pet shampoo, consider the following:

Quality
Good quality shampoos may be more expensive; however, the pet is generally bathed less frequently. A shampoo that has a lower pH than human shampoos is desirable.

Ingredients
Look for natural ingredients that are hypoallergenic, non-irritating to the eyes, repel bugs and have a nice fragrance. Chamomile and lavender are natural bug deterrents that have a pleasant smell.

Specific Needs
Some pets may require medicated shampoos for the treatment of skin disorders such as psoriasis, seborrhea and dermatitis. These products may be available over the counter or may require a prescription from the veterinarian. In some cases, these products are applied to the pet and left on for a prescribed amount of time before being rinsed.

Flea and tick shampoos contain chemicals such as pyrethrin and permethrin that kill fleas and ticks but are not irritating to the pets' skin. These products are generally safe for most pets, but some are not designed for use in very young animals. Pyrethrins are organic compounds naturally derived from the Chrysanthemum flower. They are non-persistent, biodegradable, and break down with exposure to light or oxygen. Permethrin is a synthetic chemical with similar efficacy as an insecticide.

Some shampoos are designed to enhance the pets' coat, making it shinier and looking great. Some shampoos have color additives and whiteners to enhance the pets' natural coat.

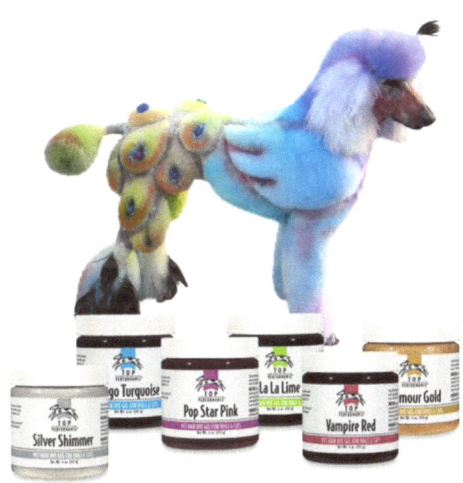

Medicated Dips
Unlike shampoos that clean and deodorize, medicated dips are designed to treat specific ailments without being rinsed off the pet. Some dips are designed to treat skin disease and infection, while others are used as insecticides. Medicated dips can be used to treat flea infestations and mange mites. These products are generally potent concentrates that

require dilution before being applied to the pet. Additionally, they may be irritating to the skin of grooming staff, making safety equipment such as gloves and eye protection essential when working with these products.

Other Grooming Procedures

In addition to baths and dips, pets may require additional procedures while at the grooming facility. Matted hair, long nails and pet scooting may be quickly remedied by the groomer.

Mats

Hair matting can be an indicator of illness and a lack of grooming by the pet, and can harbor foreign material leading to discomfort to the pet. Mats may be combed out using a wire pet comb; however, care should be taken not to pull too vigorously causing unnecessary pain to the pet. Electric hair clippers are an easy and safe method of mat removal on a pet, because it is not necessary to pull the mat, and there is little risk of cutting the skin. Scissors should not be used for clipping mats because inadvertent cutting of the pet's skin can occur.

Ear Cleaning

Ear cleaning may include flushing of the ear canals as well as the removal of hair within the canal. In some pets, such as toy breeds, the accumulation of ear canal hair can limit the ears ability to maintain dryness, leading to yeast, fungal and bacterial infections. A small hemostat can be used to remove the canal hair in these breeds, although it can cause some discomfort, so care should be taken. Clipping the underside of the ear flap or pinna, can also help increase airflow to the canal.

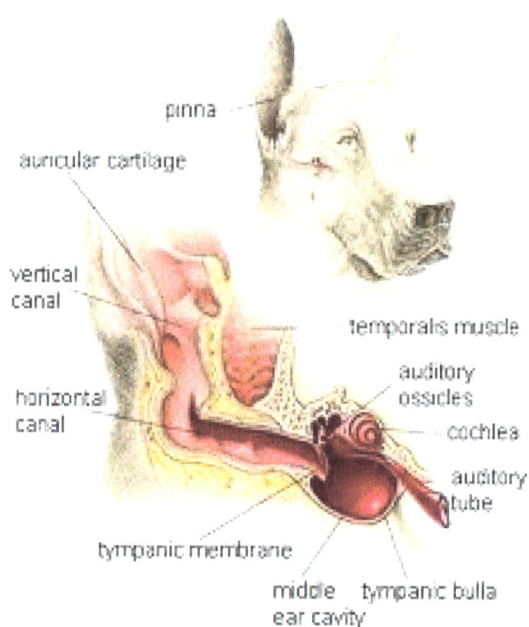

Figure 127: Anatomy of the dog ear

Ear canal flushing is designed to loosen and remove ear wax and debris from within the canal. These liquid products contain emulsifiers and astringents that break up wax and help dry the canal quickly. Ear flushing generally involves the filling of the entire canal with the cleaning solution. Gentle massaging of the base of the ear will help loosen debris deep within the ear canal. Care should be taken not to massage the ear base too vigorously as this can lead to a temporary paresis of the facial nerves called Horner's Syndrome. A towel can be used to cover the pet's head once the cleaning solution has been instilled. A pet will frequently shake their head vigorously; this forces both the cleaning solution and debris out of the canals. The towel provides a barrier from the ensuing liquid spray. After the ears have been cleaned, a gentle wiping with cotton or a soft towel will remove excess liquid and debris from within the canal and the inside of the pinna. Care should be taken when using cotton tipped applicators deep in the ear canal, although, due to the anatomy of dog and cat ear, it would be difficult to traumatize the tympanic membrane or ear canal. The surface of the ear canal is delicate and can be injured with improper use of cotton tipped applicators. Ear cleanings are generally done based on external observations of ear debris, or because of odors within the canal. Cleanings may be done frequently, but chronic ear debris and odor may be indicative of a more serious ear problem such as infection, or a foreign body that will require veterinary intervention.

Nail Trimming

Overgrown nails can be a problem for both pets and their owners. Long nails can be uncomfortable for pets and sharp nails can ruin furniture or cause scratches including those that lead to the zoonotic disease cat scratch fever. Nail trimming can be a painless and quick procedure, however, some pets are not accustom to the act and can make things very challenging. It is recommended that pet owners desensitize their pets for nail trimming at an early age; this could save valuable time and money.

The equipment necessary for effective nail trimming includes a pair of sharp nail trimmers such as the Resco guillotine style trimmers. Additionally, a blood clotting styptic powder will be useful in the event of an inadvertent cutting of the nails' blood supply, commonly called the quick.

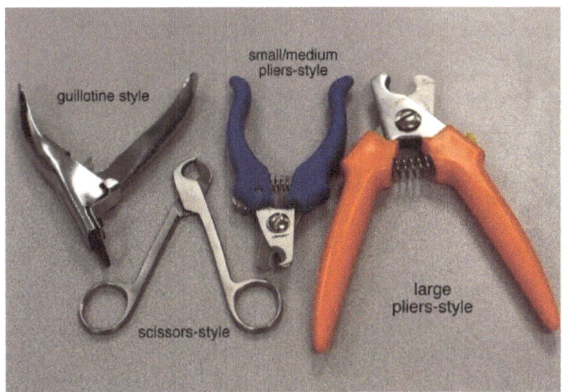

Figure 128: Assorted nail trimmers

The nail originates from the germinal tissue of the third phalanx of each digit in most species of animals. In dogs and cats, as well as other animals that walk on their toes, overgrown nails can cause discomfort in the digits if left unmanaged. In most cases, the daily act of walking and running on hard surfaces wears down the nails naturally. Animals not utilizing these surfaces, being inactive or because of illness, may lead them to overgrown nails. Horses, for example, need regular hoof trimming to maintain the length and articulation of their nails. The nail in all species has a blood supply, or 'quick', that nourishes the growing nail. Trimming requires the understanding of where the quick is located, and how long the nail should be. In dogs and cats, as well as many species of animal, walking is a result of standing on one's toes. Nails need to be shorter than the pad or digit in order to prevent discomfort. If a tangential line is drawn from the pad, the nail should not exceed that plane.

Many animals have semi-transparent nails, while others have dark, opaque nails. Those with semi-transparent nails have visible quicks that are easily identifiable; the dark nailed animals are more challenging. Relying on the tangential line and a notch on the underside of the nail of many species,

103

an accurate nail trim can be accomplished. The nail should be cut at a forty-five degree angle from the tangential line and nail notch, if present. In some animals, the quick will be longer than thought, and bleeding from the nail may occur and can be painful to the pet. The use of styptic powder will effectively stop the bleeding if this occurs. Some veterinary practices pack styptic powder into a syringe case for use, while others use moistened cotton tipped applicators.

Nail cross section

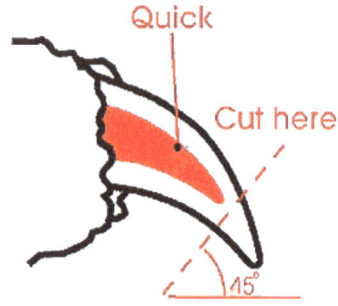

Figure 129: Diagram showing nail trimming location and angle

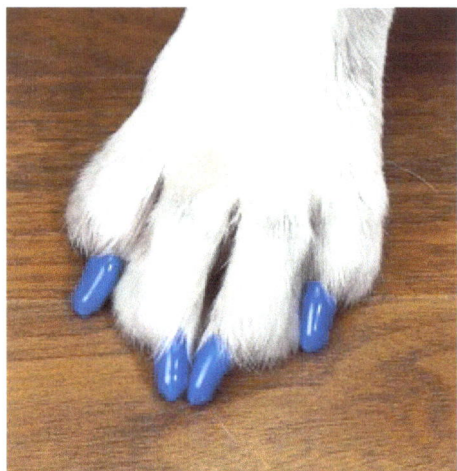

Figure 130: Cosmetic nail colors and covers for pets

Anal Sac Expression

The anal sacs function to scent feces as it is leaving the rectum. This powerful olfactant communicates information to other animals, and in many cases, helps define territorial boundaries. Some animals will express their anal glands when stressed or frightened. Anal gland secretions are brownish and very pungent. The anal glands are located at four and eight o'clock on the rectal opening. Under normal circumstances, the passing of feces forces out anal gland material, scenting that material as it passes. If the glands become infected or impacted with material, or the pet has diarrhea, the anal glands may impact and become irritated. The first sign of this irritation is the classic "scooting" observed by many pet owners. Once expressed, the scooting likely resolves; under extreme circumstances, surgical removal of the anal glands may be necessary.

Using a gloved hand, lubricate the first digit with KY jelly or a similar lubricant and insert the digit into the anal opening. Using a smaller digit like the 'pinkie' may be beneficial when expressing the anal glands of very small animals. With the digit fully inserted into the anus, begin to curl the finger back towards the anal opening, (at four or eight o'clock), making contact with the inner anal wall. As the digit begins to leave the anus, any gland material will be expressed out onto the gloved hand. Clean the perianal area with a mild soap and water, followed by any grooming spray to provide a pleasant scent.

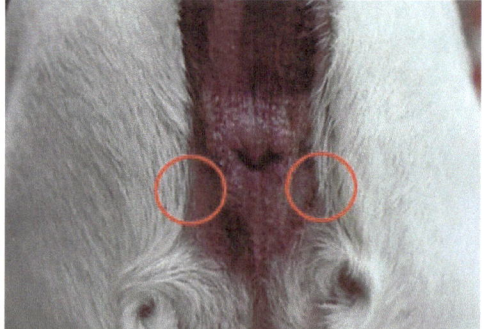

Figure 131: Location of anal glands in animals

104

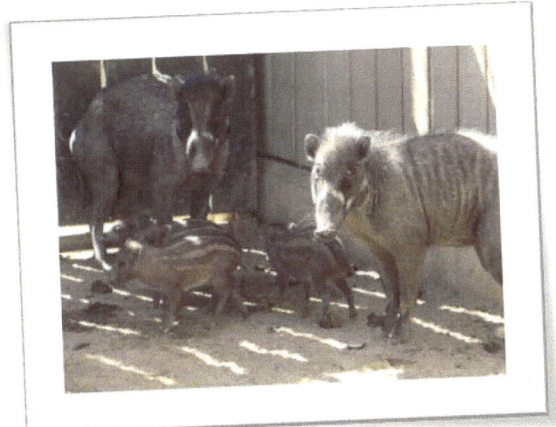

Figure 132: Visayan warty pigs

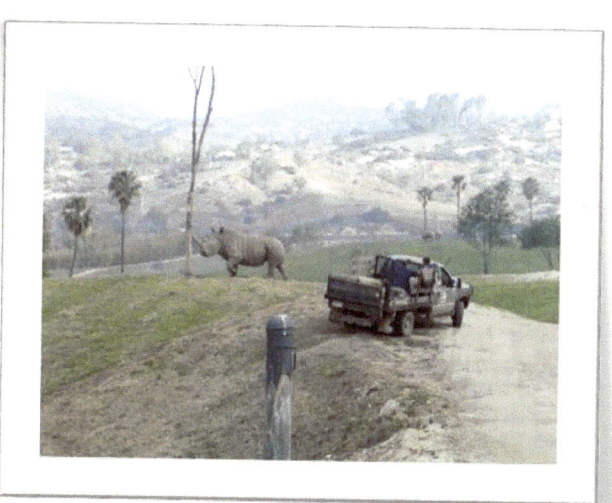

Figure 133: Southern white rhinoceros immobilization

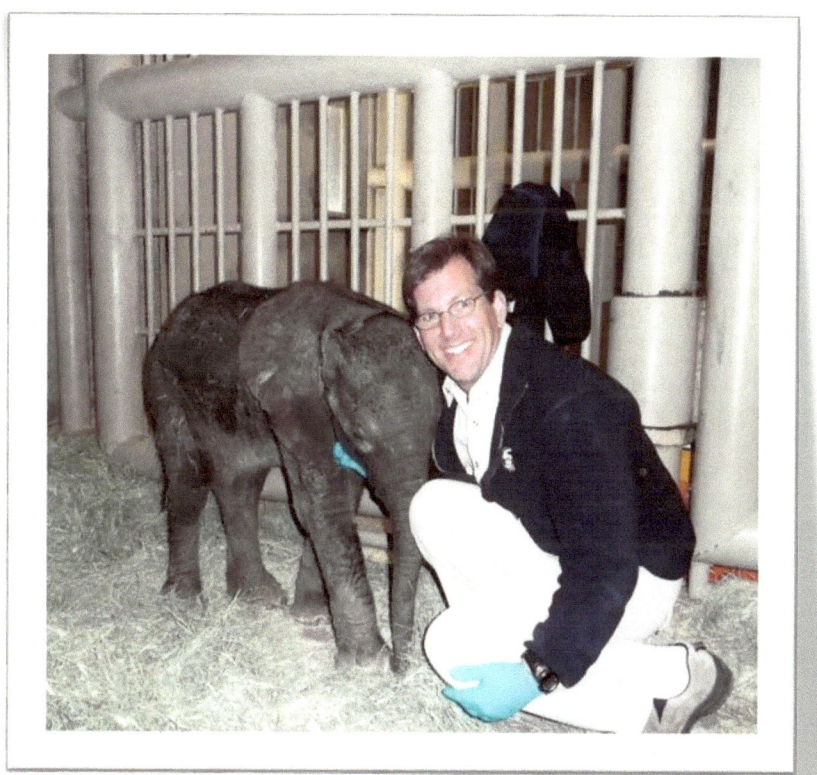

Figure 134: African elephant calf

New Technologies

Technological advances are developing at an amazing pace. Film cameras have been quickly replaced by their digital counterparts, and computer advances have afforded advances in digital data acquisition and storage. Electronic medical record systems and digital image capture have enabled users the ability to send information and images quickly to specialists across the country. Advances in equipment, procedures and medications have improved animal diagnosis and care. Work with genes and stem cells will continue to propel medicine forward at an astonishing rate.

Ultrasound

Developed from SONAR technology, ultrasound uses sound waves to penetrate the body and generate images based on the refraction of the sound. SONAR, stands for SOund, Navagation And Ranging, and is used by the military to identify ships and submarines in water. Sound travels farther in water than air; because animal bodies are made up of primarily water, sonar sound waves transmit well through them.

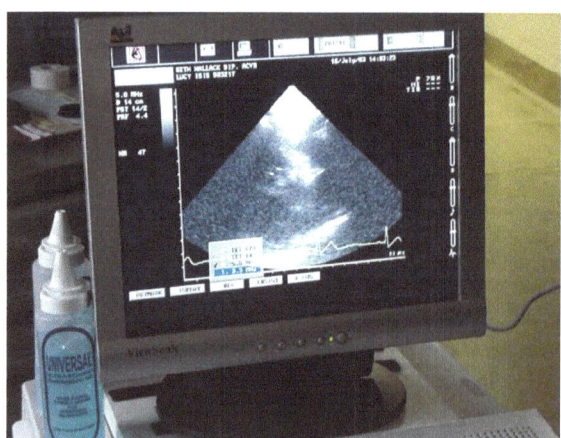

Figure 135: A cardiac ultrasound image of an anteater

Flow Doppler

Flow Doppler interprets blood flow direction in an ultrasound image. The Doppler concept originates from the astronomy principle that celestial bodies that are moving towards you will have higher energy associated with them when compared to those objects when they are moving away. Lower energy is cooler and appears bluish when viewing stars, while those moving towards us appear more reddish. This principle enables ultrasound users to see blood flow moving away from the probe (blue) as well as blood flow moving towards the probe (red).

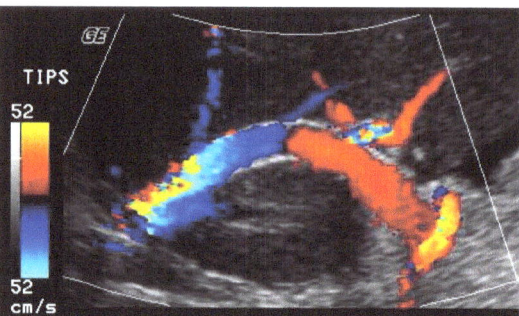

Figure 136: Ultrasound image using doppler

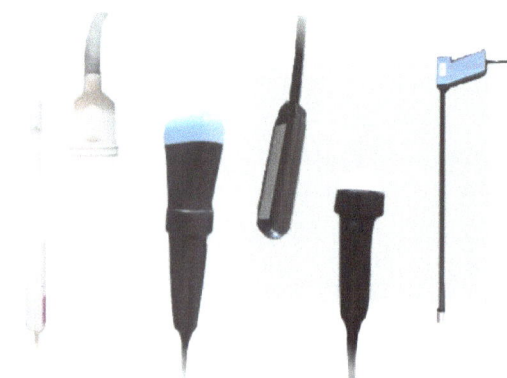

Figure 137: Assorted ultrasound probes

X-ray Modalities

X-ray imaging is a valuable diagnostic resource in veterinary medicine. Diagnostic radiology and the advent of digital image capture systems have revolutionized the way x-ray images are viewed, stored and shared. X-rays are also useful in diagnosing and treating some kinds of tumors or enabling surgeons to see 'real time' images taken intra-operatively.

Diagnostic Radiology

The mainstay of most veterinary practices, the radiographic images obtained is used for diagnosis of diseases or fractures. The images are black and white, with shades of grey. Ideally suited for images of bone, x-rays, when used correctly, can also show organs and soft tissue with significant clarity.

Digital Radiography

Digital radiology has further enhanced diagnostic radiographs by improving image quality, clarity and versatility. By use of a computer, captured images can have adjustments made to image contrast and magnification. Images can be easily sent to specialists via e-mail and stored in image vaults instead of filing cabinets. Most systems are standardized in a DICOM (digital imaging and communications in medicine) format, enabling most users to open and view images easily.

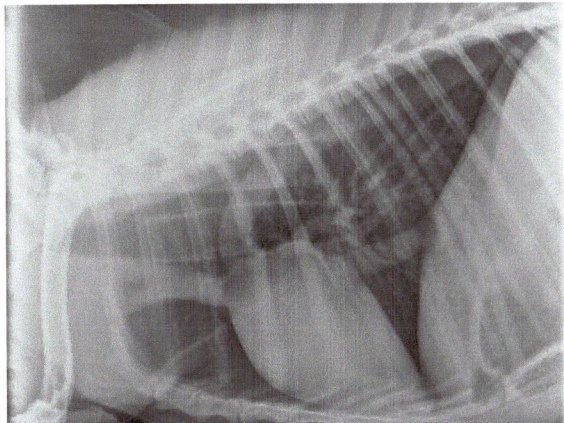

Figure 138: Digital chest radiograph: note clarity of image, presence of aortic arch, coronary artery and bronchioles

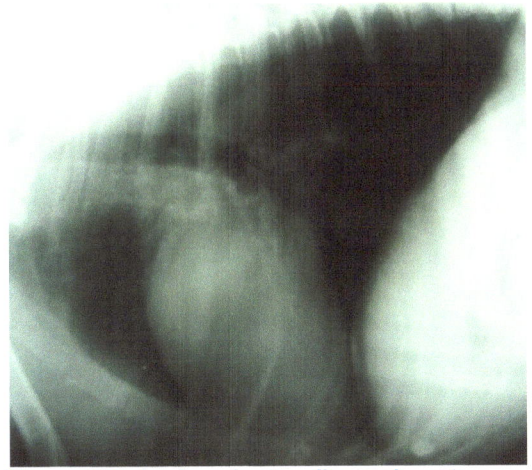

Figure 139: Analog chest radiograph; note reduced detail when compared to digital image

Fluoroscopy

Also called 'real time' radiology, uses lower energy x-rays to obtain live images of the patient. Fluoroscopy is commonly used during angioplasty, but can be useful in retrieving vascular foreign bodies, determining disc space positioning and cystogram placement.

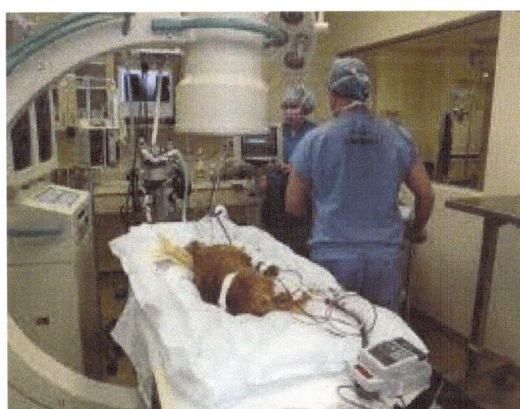

Figure 140: Fluoroscope

Scintigraphy (Nuclear Medicine)

Scintigraphy uses gamma radiation cameras and radionuclides to identify organ function or metastatic bone lesions in patients. The radionuclide most commonly used is Technetium 99m. Scintigraphy can diagnose organ function and ailments earlier than other modalities.

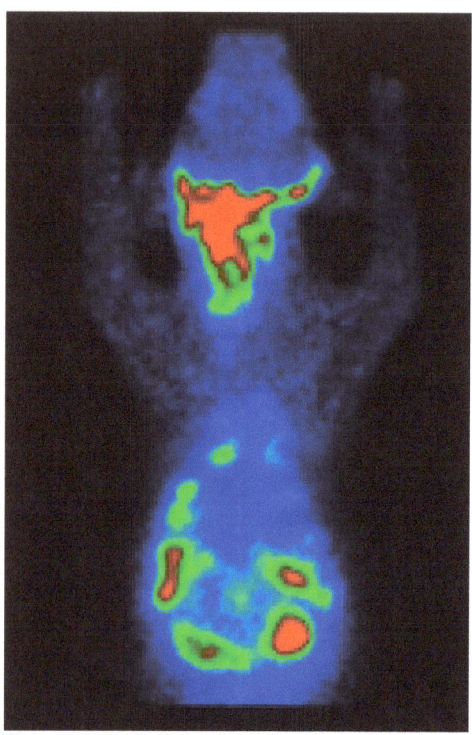

Figure 141: Scintograph image of a dog

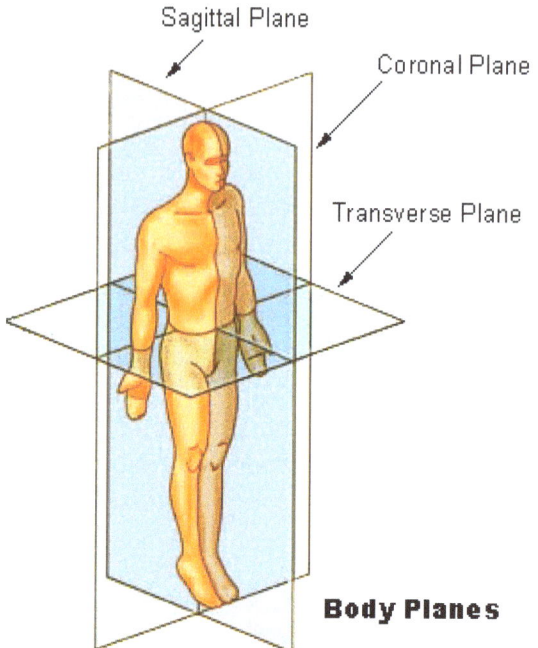

Figure 142: Diagram of the body planes used in CT and MRI studies

Computed Axial Tomography (CAT)

CT scans or CAT scans use x-rays to produce image 'slices' or tomographic images of predetermined areas of a patient. The slices that are generated may be a centimeter or as small as a millimeter apart. CT studies require significantly more x-ray exposure to the patient, and potentially more exposure to the technician. Ultimately, CT scans are beneficial in determining injuries to bone, lung and chest studies and tumor formation. CT scans are more cost effective and tend to be utilized in emergency situations because a scan may only take five minutes.

In general, the slices that CT generates can be from one of three planes. The most common image is generated in the transverse plane. It slices the body from top to bottom, or in animals, from front to back. The other slices that can be imaged include the sagittal and coronal planes. Sagittal images are useful in spinal cord studies and images of the brain.

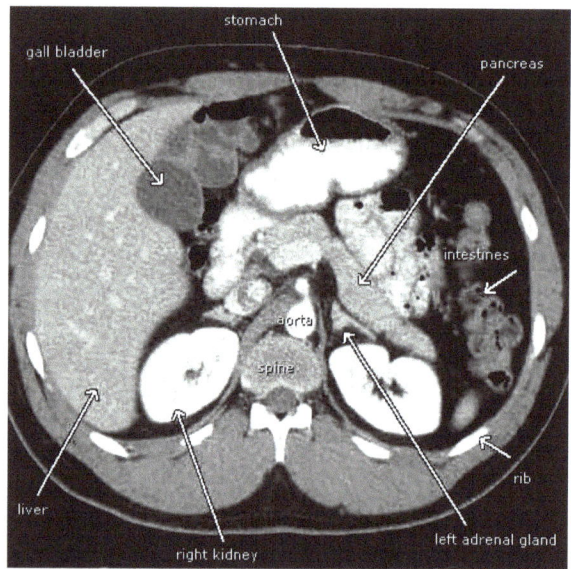

Figure 143: A transverse CT image showing several organs, spine and ribs

Get a candy bar. Picture what a slice of it looks like. Cut the candy bar in half and see if it looks like what you thought it would.

108

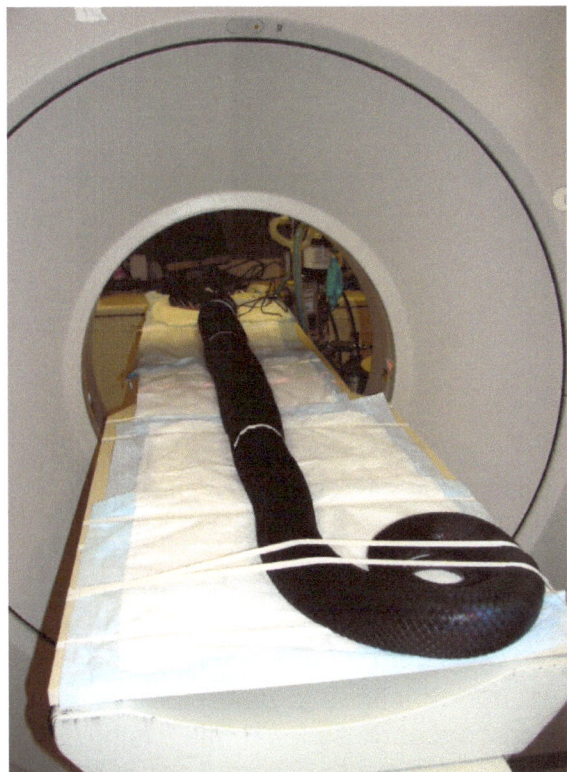
Figure 144: Boelens python in CT unit

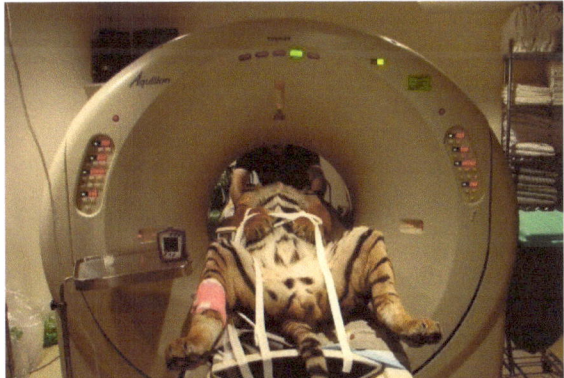
Figure 145: Indochinese Tiger getting a CT of his skull

Magnetic Resonance Imagery (MRI)

MRI technology utilizes a magnet to change and measure the polarity movements of hydrogen atoms in the body. Hydrogen can be found in water (H_2O) and makes up a significant part of all bio-organisms. The resultant 'slices' are similar to those of CT scans. Images are generally made in the transverse plane. MRI units are longer than CT units; the patient is in a tunnel rather than a doughnut.

MRI is ideally suited for soft tissue exams such as tendons, ligaments, spinal cord as well as brain injuries. Scans may take thirty minutes or more. It is important that all metal be removed from the patient, operators and the room prior to a scan. When anesthetized for MRI's, animal patients require special anesthetic machines and oxygen tanks that are not magnet attractants. Unlike CT units, veterinary support staff may be in the MRI suite when imaging is taking place without occupational hazard. MRI units will, however, deactivate most credit cards and other cards with magnetic strips. Belts, earrings and other piercings should be removed prior to entering a MRI suite. The noise of a MRI unit can be loud; ear protection for veterinary support may be necessary.

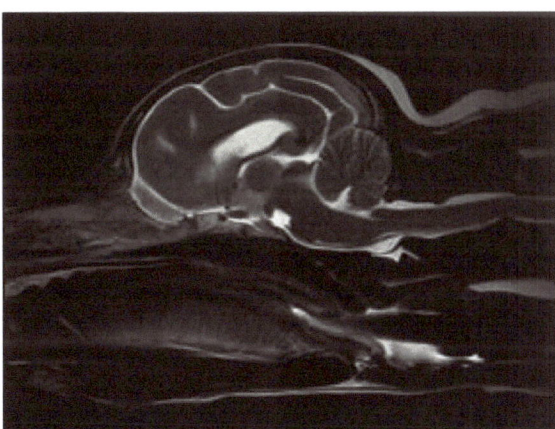
Figure 146: Sagittal view of a dog skull and brain with MRI imagery

Thermal Imagery

Thermal imagery makes use of the heat signature emitted by all organisms. Infection and inflammation causes localized heating; as a result, thermal imaging may help diagnose early joint injuries and infections before they are overtly apparent. This technology may be beneficial to animals that are large, or cannot be readily handled or restrained for examination.

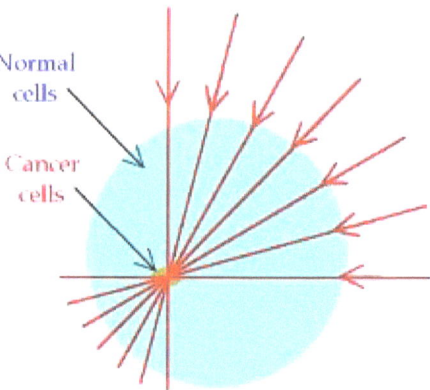

Figure 148: Diagram of radiotherapy use in tumor eradication and treatment

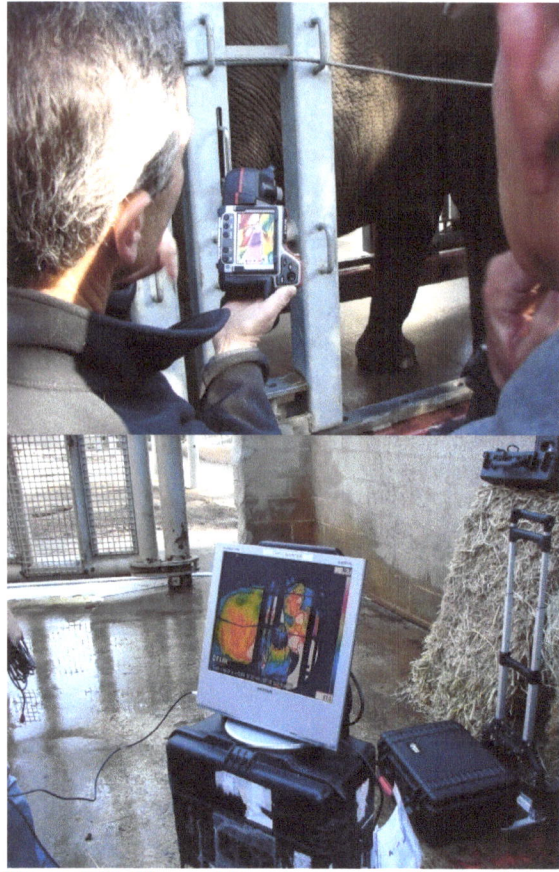

Figure 147: Thermal imaging camera (top) and resultant image of an elephant

Radiotherapy

Radiotherapy, also known as radiation therapy, utilizes high energy radiation (gamma rays) to destroy cancer cells. It is often used in conjunction with traditional chemotherapies. The radiation damages DNA responsible for the replication of malignant tumor cells, thus, eliminating proliferation of these cells. Ideally, the tumor is exposed to a larger absorbed radiation dose than the surrounding tissue leading to eradication of the tumor cells.

Stem Cells

Somatic stem cells are the precursor cells of the cellular constituents of blood. Stem cells from bone marrow have been used for decades to treat blood disorders such as leukemia. Using compatible marrow from a donor, stem cells can be injected into a patient; normal blood cells are then produced by the donor's stem cells.

In recent years, stem cell rich umbilical cords have been used to treat those diseases treated with the more invasive bone marrow procedure. Umbilical cord stem cells are less prone to rejection by the patient.

Today, precursor cells from other tissues, such as adipose, have yielded undifferentiated cells, that when properly targeted, have been used to treat diseases including autism, cerebral palsy, arthritis, multiple sclerosis, heart disease and spinal cord injuries. These stem cells attempt to replace damaged or degenerative tissue cells, and in some cases, repair the site of damage. Much of this work is being done outside of the US in countries such as Panama, because of FDA regulatory hurdles.

In animals, stem cells are being used to treat arthritis and injuries associated with lameness. As this procedure gains popularity for pet owners, it is important to recognize its limitations:

- Stem cells are tissue specific; the precursor cells that produce blood cannot at this time make heart and nerve cells.
- Results may vary and be subtle; many treatments may be needed to produce any effect.
- Even when using a patient's own stem cells, there is a risk of rejection as well as infection associated with the procedure.
- The collection, culture and cultivation of stem cells is a laborious process.

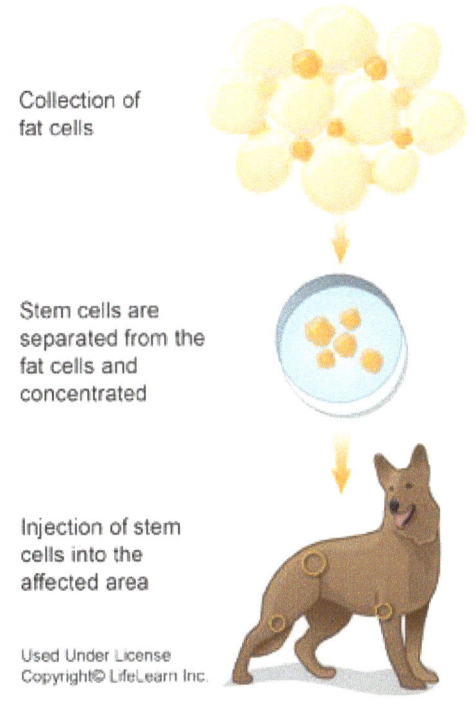

Collection of fat cells

Stem cells are separated from the fat cells and concentrated

Injection of stem cells into the affected area

Figure 149: General concept of stem cell use in animals

Cloning

Cloning, or the identical replication of an individual, is seen as a good method for the production of agricultural animals such as cows, pigs, goats and sheep.

Cloning, or the identical replication of an individual, is seen as a good method for the production of agricultural animals such as cows, pigs, goats and sheep. As an attempt to curb extinction, cloning is thought to be a viable method to preserve and propagate endangered species. As in the movie Jurassic Park, viable DNA from an extinct species may be used to produce a living specimen. The process of cloning requires a donor egg cell and viable DNA from the animal to be cloned. Donor DNA is replaced with DNA from animal being cloned. Viable egg is then incubated in a surrogate individual until parturition. The resultant offspring is identical phenotypically and genotypically to the animal being cloned. Challenges to cloning include:

- Stress placed on donor egg cell and nucleus during DNA transfer is substantial leading to high cell loss.
- Survivability of embryos is low.
- The insertion of DNA is not automated and must be done manually using a microscope, making it time consuming and expensive.
- The biochemistry of cell activation has not been fully understood or mastered.

111

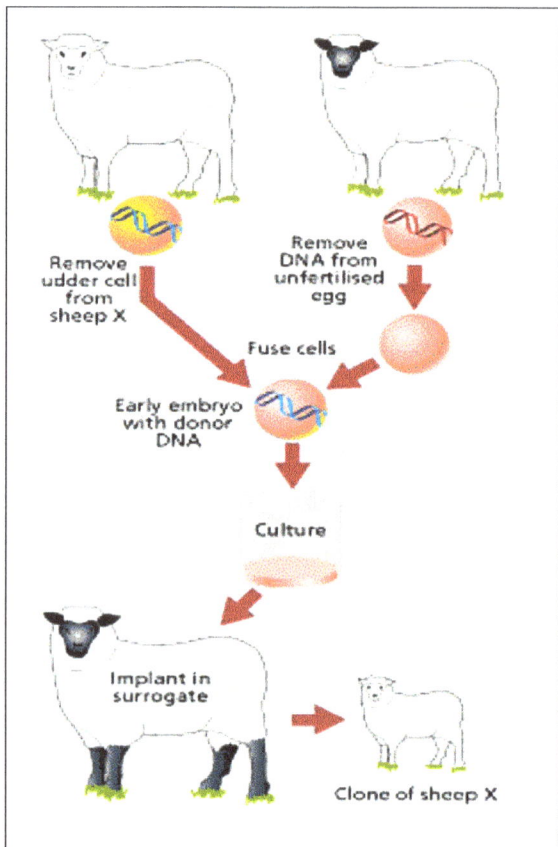

Figure 150: Diagram showing process of cloning

Cryobanking

Tissue samples, eggs and sperm can be preserved indefinitely in ultra-cold freezers. Liquid nitrogen can be used to super freeze these samples without damage. Liquid nitrogen freezers can maintain temperatures of less than minus 350 degrees Fahrenheit. Cryobanking is not new, first stored from livestock since the 1950's; it is now recognized as a means to store samples for conservation purposes. Both animal and plant specimens have been cryobanked for future use and propagation. The term 'frozen zoo' has been used to describe animal cell samples stored by exotic animal and zoo institutions.

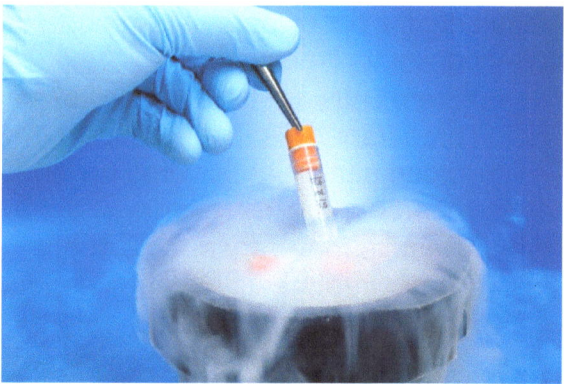

Figure 151: Samples are stored in cryo containers

Surgery

Advances in surgery, surgical techniques and instrumentation have made surgery more efficient, effective and often times, less invasive. New surgical techniques and equipment have revolutionized traditional surgical practices.

Electrocautery

Electrocautery, also known as thermal cautery, uses electrical current to cause tissue destruction. It is commonly used as a scalpel, creating an incision in tissue without bleeding. Cauterization seals blood vessels and reduces blood loss associated with surgery. Electrocautery probes are metal tipped and shaped like a wand or thumb forceps.

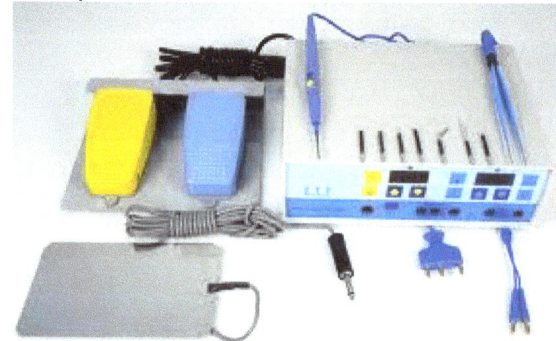

Figure 152: Electro-cauterization unit

CO₂ Lasers

Carbon Dioxide (CO_2) lasers are used in surgery as a scalpel much like electrocautery. They are also used for less invasive procedures such as dermabrasion and skin resurfacing. CO_2 lasers produce a beam of infrared light capable of cutting or destroying tissue, while being well absorbed by water; a major component of tissues.

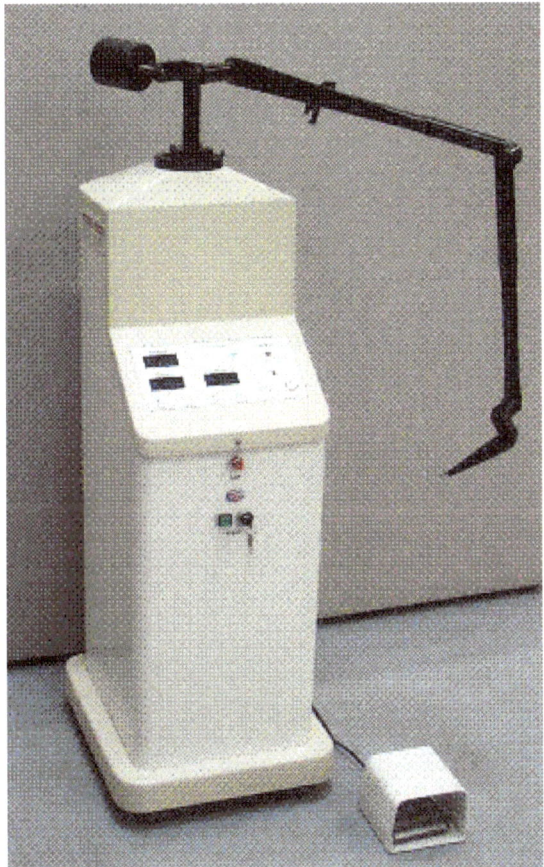

Figure 153: CO_2 laser

Microsurgery

Microsurgery is a general term for surgery requiring small instruments and in some cases a microscope. Microsurgeries have allowed surgeons to perform anastomosis or connect small vessels together, enabling the ability to repair vessel damage as well as facilitate organ transplantation. Corneal transplant and other ophthalmic procedures require the use of microsurgery.

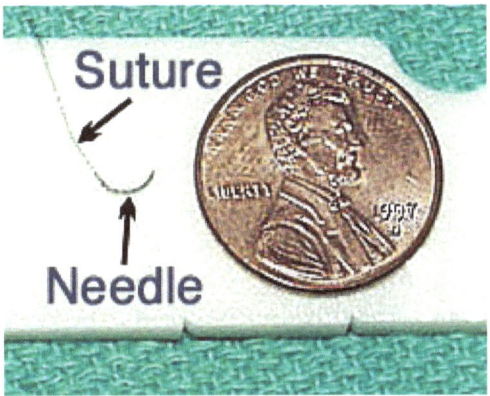

Figure 154: Microsurgery suture

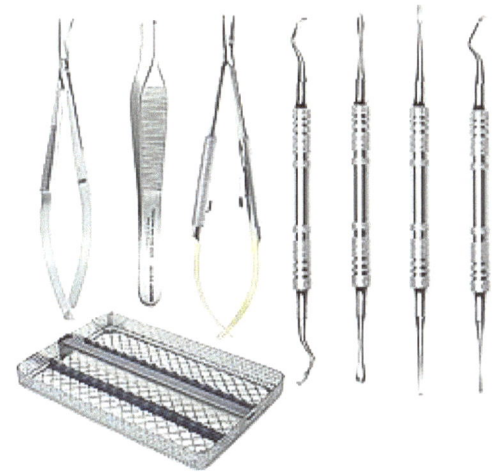

Figure 155: Common microsurgical instruments

Endoscopy

Endoscopy has revolutionized surgery and surgical recovery time by reducing incision size and patient post operative care. In people, endoscopy is now used for procedures like cholecystectomies, (gall bladder removal), appendectomies and hysterectomies. Knee and shoulder surgery is also facilitated with an endoscope. In animals, endoscopy is used to visualize the stomach (gastroscopy) or view the nasal passages and lungs (bronchoscopy). Endoscopes have a fiber optic viewing system, an eyepiece or camera attachment, as well as a powerful light source to illuminate the internal structures of the body. Most endoscopes also have a channel in which grabbing tools or cutters may be passed into the body.

Types of endoscopes include:

- Laparoscope-a rigid scope used to look into the abdomen. It is often used to look for gonads in bird species for gender determination.
- Arthroscope-a rigid scope much like the laparoscope, but used to look into joint spaces such as the knee.
- Flexible endoscope-an endoscope capable of bending with the use of directional dials. These scopes are commonly used for gastric and digestive studies where curves and corners are common.

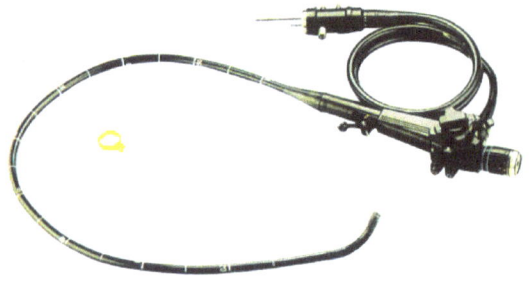

Figure 157: Flexible endoscope

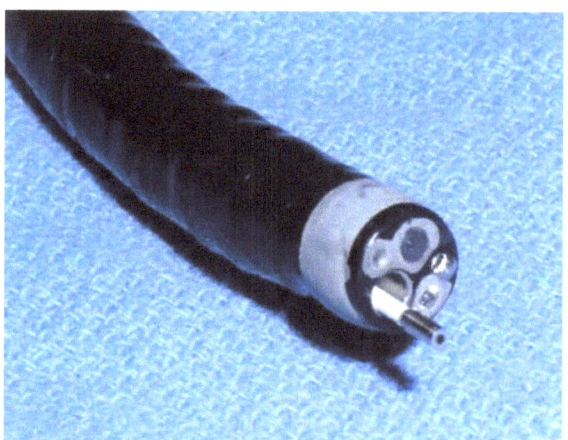

Figure 158: Flexible endoscope showing light source and instrument cannula

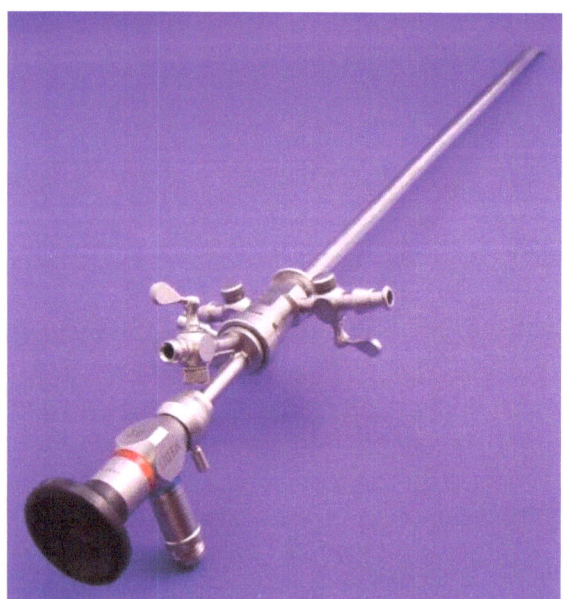

Figure 156: A typical laparoscope with cannula

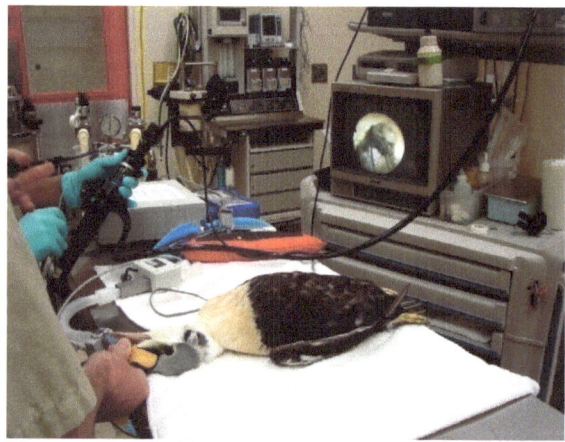

Figure 159: Flexible endoscopy of a King Eider

Conclusion

You now have all of the tools necessary to work with exotic animals, and if you read my companion animal "essentials", you have acquired everything that I have used in my career to become a proficient veterinary professional. There are still challenges ahead, let's face it, we live in a competitive world; you, however, now have a competitive edge. Here are a few additional suggestions to become even more competitive:

- Get hands on experience
  - You will gain confidence and experience working with assorted exotic species.
  - You will see how exotic animals behave.
- Get an exotic pet
  - There is no better way to understand animal handling and husbandry than to maintain a healthy pet; be prepared for a commitment and research the exotic you may be interested in. Only obtain a legal exotic from a reputable pet store; don't take animals from the wild.
- Volunteer
  - Find a wildlife rehabilitation facility, zoo, farm, research facility or pet store and volunteer your time; this is a great way to get experience and allow potential employers see your dedication and work ethic.

Everyone has the ability to attain their dream! Hard work and confidence is the key..I can't stress that enough. Good luck in your desire to be a veterinary professional!

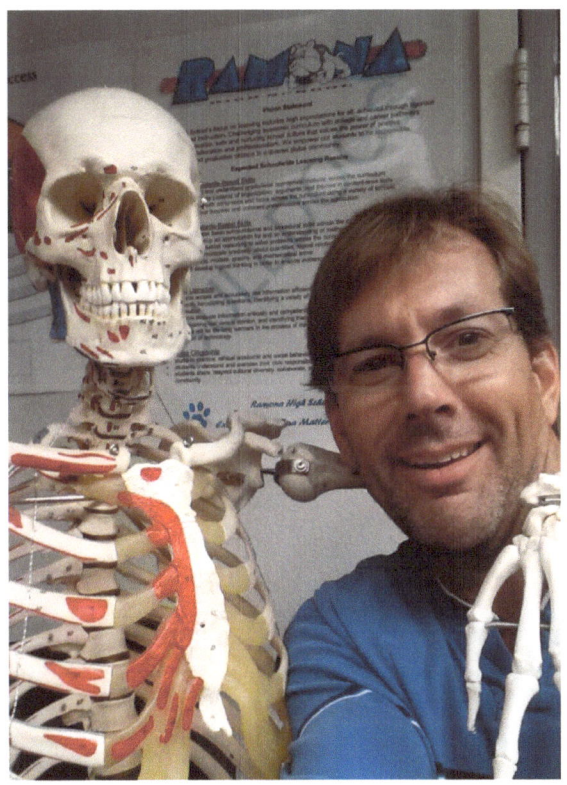

www.ingramcontent.com/pod-product-compliance
Lightning Source LLC
Chambersburg PA
CBHW050724180526
45159CB00003B/1123